Kristin

I remember you well from ART and the ALC — I appreciate your work with adolescents! Tough group for sure. Enjoy — you will be able to relate

TARGET PRACTICE

*Twelve Years in the Trenches
and the Counselor in Recovery*

Tim Volz

Started in March 2016

ISBN: 978-1-66785-993-4

CONTENTS

PART VI

Review for *Target Practice*

"I didn't know the difference between someone who is sober and someone who is in recovery. Actually, I didn't know there was a difference until I read this book.

When I needed help for a family member who overdosed on drugs, I reached out to those I knew that ran recovery centers. Tim put action behind his words and immediately jumped into our boat to help us row out of the turbulent waters we'd found ourselves in.

Simply put, Tim Volz is a man of action, compassion and empathy who digs in to help when others just point you in a direction to get help.

The gifts he's gained while walking through the system as an addict, recovering addict and now counselor of addicts give him the credibility to write this book which should be read by all who struggle with a drug or alcohol problem. Why? Because as you'll read, the information he's gathered through tough experience is followed up with education and training that makes him an insightful expert.

Not only do I highly recommend this book, I will have several copies on hand to personally give to people when I know they need help."

Betsy Singer
Broadcast Journalist

Foreword to *Target Practice*

Tim has written a book of two journeys. First, Tim shares his journey through his own addiction, how it began, how it progressed, and finally how, with honesty, humility, and tenacity, he found a sustained recovery, a recovery he does not take for granted, a recovery that requires continuing care and attention. The reader has no doubt that Tim understands addiction and recovery from the inside out.

Tim shares his second journey as a professional in the world of recovery. The challenges are different but very real. Tim has worked in several treatment settings gaining in-depth knowledge and experience in the process. He has seen firsthand the flaws in the current system. As I read the book, I was concerned that a reader might look at Tim's moves from program to program and conclude that he is a malcontent who is never satisfied. That conclusion would be incorrect. Tim's moves provided opportunities to practice his profession in the way he believed it should be practiced. Tim is not willing to accept the status quo when he knows there is a better way.

Tim is not alone in offering critiques of the current treatment of addiction. Many experts agree. A recent review of current research on the treatment of addiction revealed wide-spread concern regarding gaps in the treatment of addiction. The term "gaps" has been used to describe weak points in the system that result in sub-optimal care. In spite of the costs (social, emotional, physical, psychological, and financial) associated with addiction for individuals, families, and society, treatment for many is insufficient and fragmented. Despite an increased understanding of the disease of addiction and evidence of effective strategies for treatment, substantial gaps persist.

The gaps Tim described from his personal perspective and the gaps described in the professional literature from the scientific perspective are similar. In his book, Tim has provided practical insight into the same gaps identified by researchers.

Experts describe a "treatment gap," in which only about 12 % of persons who need treatment for addiction actually receive treatment. The reasons for this are complex and multifaceted but one of the most significant contributors is an inability to afford appropriate treatment. Professionals conduct a comprehensive assessment and make a recommendation for the treatment that is needed but it is insurance companies that often decide the treatment a person gets. Tim often provides the care that is needed irrespective of payment (or lack thereof). This may not be a sustainable business model if profit is the goal, but it is a model that leads to sustained recovery for his clients.

A second major cause of the "treatment gap" is the client's ambivalence to engage in treatment. Tim helps clients to discover within themselves the motivation to get better......then he shows them how. His approach is person-centered and holistic. He reaches out with integrity, authenticity, and willingness to meet people where they are. Once he commits to a client, he doesn't give up easily. The client may walk away from Tim, but Tim doesn't walk away from a client who is willing to try. His willingness to believe in their recovery sends a powerful message to those who have not yet learned to believe in themselves.

A second major gap relates to persons with a dual diagnosis. Approximately 50% of persons with addiction also have a mental health disorder. Evidence is clear that both conditions need to be treated if the client is to recover from either. However, treatment for both is often the exception rather than the rule in part because most professionals are qualified to treat one and not the other, making integrated treatment challenging. Licensed drug and alcohol counselors are often not qualified to treat mental health disorders. Conversely, mental health counselors may lack the qualifications to treat addiction. In his book, Tim describes how, at a significant personal and financial cost, Tim pursued education and licensure in both areas so that he could offer integrated treatment as supported by scientific evidence.

Persons with addiction are often victims of the "continuity of care" gap, a gap that allows persons to fall through the cracks, especially at times of transition. Tim addressed this gap by providing long-term group and individual treatment...and continuing that support when treatment was interrupted by relapse, residential treatment, detox, or hospitalization. Tim was also instrumental in increasing opportunities for medication-assisted treatment, another strategy strongly supported by research.

Tim conducts regular family support groups which are very helpful. But more importantly, he has been able to forge a partnership with families and work with families on how best to support their loved one. Tim makes family members feel part of the solution, not part of the problem.

I know many competent, compassionate, and committed treatment professionals, and yet, Tim is unique and a bit of a maverick. Tim is known as one of the most effective and respected treatment providers in our community. He also consults with programs throughout the state. The system needs change and Tim's book has provided insight into the changes that are needed. Some look at the shortcomings of the current system for treating addiction and ask, "Why?" Tim looks for innovative solutions and asks, "Why not?" Tim is a critical thinker, willing to challenge old ways of thinking. Tim actively seeks new ideas and new ways of solving old problems. I am hopeful that it will be thinkers and innovators like Tim who will help lead us out of the unprecedented epidemic of addiction we are now enduring.

Gayle Olsen, MS, CNP

President, Board of Directors

Community Pathways to Family Health and Recovery

"You have enemies? Good. That means you stood up for something, sometime in your life." - Winston Churchill,

"When you lose everything, and I mean everything, you sit there in this empty room in the dark, and the only person who can get you out is you. The hardest thing in life to do is to change." – Mickey Rourke.

Target Practice—
The Meaning of the Title and Other Notes

I want the reader to know a couple of things before you get started reading the book. First and foremost, I live a life of recovery today, which means a lot of different things to a lot of different people. For some people, like my clients, I imagine I am someone to look up to. Some of my current and past colleagues see my personal experience and education as an asset to an organization, and they value both. There is also a third group of people, and it is hard to explain who these folks are. They do not appear to be big fans of the counselor in recovery. They might have worked with a counselor in recovery and had a bad experience. They might have seen a counselor in recovery make poor decisions with clients in the past. They might not agree with some of the methods of the counselor in recovery. They may be jealous of their "comeback" in life. I really don't know the exact reasons for this, but I have seen it manifest in multiple places over the 12 years I have worked in the profession. Maybe William White says it best in his book *Slaying the Dragon: The History of Addiction Treatment and Recovery* where he states that "Most professionals do not like alcoholics and addicts." I have had people attack me personally many times in my career (always after I leave a facility), and it has benefited me greatly to work a strong recovery program, or this would have eaten me up. There is a big difference between a counselor who is sober and a counselor who is in recovery. I have seen many people in recovery pursue counseling degrees and then stop working their own personal programs. If I had done that, I would not have been able to endure this twelve-year stint. For example, I have built up a lot of resentments while in the addiction counseling field, and I had to work very hard to let them go and find some peace. It was hard to relive some of these things in the book without feeling some of the pain. I have worked hard to let go of past ruminations and bitterness, but at times, the hurt still shows, as my emotions were all over the place when putting parts of this story on paper. "Letting go" is one of the character defects that I continue to work on every day, as continued personal growth is part of my identity of "a good man getting better." This is a book that, at times, can paint a harsh picture of the treatment profession in the area where I live and work. This is simply my experience. This is not meant to be a blanket statement about the entire treatment community or substance use disorder (SUD) treatment as a whole. There are amazing programs out there and amazing people who run them. I have worked for three great agencies, where the entire staff was treated with dignity, integrity, and professionalism. I have worked for more that were not great, and this appears to be a pattern in the small section of the world I call home. I often wonder if it is that way everywhere. There appears to be a lot of jealousy in the field, and it comes mostly from owners, which trickles down through some of their more seasoned employees. I just want to tell the story and bring awareness to people in recovery from addiction who decide to make the jump into the world of addiction counseling. Be careful what you wish for. It can be the most rewarding job in the world, or it can make your whole life unravel. Much of this has to do with the people who run the agencies and your own personal recovery program.

There are many people in the world who are "yes men, or women" and who follow the crowd. A good example of this is the folks who cleaned the toilet paper off the shelves the moment some states started locking down when the COVID virus was in its infancy stages (I wonder if some of them have yet to emerge two years later). They don't question why certain rules are in place. They just get in line and follow the herd, whether they are right or wrong. They don't question, and they don't challenge. This is fine, as every person is different. However, I am not one of those people. I want to know the reasoning behind certain decisions (many times, I wish I didn't). In retrospect, it would have been much easier to be someone who just blindly followed all the rules and just "fit in." But I just cannot do that. When something does not make sense to me, I ask why.

I have always had a strong vision of what kind of service I wanted to provide to my clients and how to get that done. For example, I strongly believe in the "window of opportunity" when someone needs help. When someone drums up the courage to walk in the door where I work to ask for help, I help them. I don't send them away and give them an appointment for three weeks down the road. This is not a yearly physical. This is life and death. Treatment centers are emergency rooms, in my opinion. When someone comes in, they need to walk out with hope. That is the medicine we provide. However, most addiction treatment centers do not run that way.

In many places, when someone comes in, they are not seen or evaluated if they don't have insurance. If they have insurance, they are sent away with an appointment card for an assessment, which is usually two or three weeks out. I would estimate that, in my experience, about half of these folks do not make this appointment. A portion of them overdose and die. Most of the time, resources such as AA pamphlets, access to recovery coaches, and phone numbers are not given to the person asking for help. I am using this example because I have always questioned why people send clients away without offering some form of help. They just shrug their shoulders and say, "This is how we do things," or "Come back when you get insurance." I question the system, and for that, I have been targeted, as you will see.

People do not like the person who questions the system. Now, I have not always done this, as early on, I was pretty naïve about this field. Recovery has given me the valuable gifts of integrity, patience, and "trying to play well with others in the sandbox." However, at some point, I lost the patience to "play nicely" with agencies that simply exist to make money and give poor care to clients. They herd clients in and out like cattle in money-hungry residential agencies. Certain places that advertise as "dual diagnosis facilities" are giving their clients one hour of Telehealth with a mental health professional over their twenty-eight-day stay. They do Diagnostic Assessments while clients are still in active withdrawal and misdiagnose them, branding them with sometimes stigmatizing labels, like borderline personality disorder. Drugs run rampant in some residential facilities, and it appears easier to find drugs in some treatment centers that on the street. The longer I worked in this field of counseling, the more I saw things that made no sense to me, but no one was questioning it. I became the guy who did that. As you read through this, I hope you see how important it is to try to effect some change in the system. That is one of the multiple goals of this book. It is to educate people in recovery who are deciding to become professionals and to allow people to use their voices in a respectful way so that we may better help those struggling with addiction. I am speaking from one small corner of the world, but if any of this resonates, I hope you will use your voice to talk about issues as they arise. I have heard multiple people over the years refer to the city where I work as "cutthroat," and most of these people have a history in the field of addictions. However, no one wants to "tip the apple cart," so to speak. I read the book, *Inside Rehab* by Anne Fletcher when I was about ninety percent through with the writing for this book, and although I don't necessarily agree with everything in the book, she nails a lot of the same subjects I do. That was my cue to leave some of the travesties of justice in here as if it is happening all over the United States; it is important to talk about.

This is a book in four main parts. The first section chronicles my using, addict life, and the progression of my addiction, which is fraught with consequences, absurdities, and sadness. Yes, another memoir. However, I need to tell the reader how I got to this place, as I certainly did not grow up wanting to be a drug and alcohol counselor (I wanted to be a baseball player and then a coach). The second section details my road to recovery, including humbling stepping-stones that set up my career as a professional. It also bleeds into the next section, which includes some personal road-blocks in my career and how I was able to work through those barriers. The third section is the state of the counseling profession (in my humble experience), the extra pressure of the counselor in recovery, and what my recovery looks like today. It also offers potential solutions, from my perspective. The last section emphasizes the importance of educating the counselor in recovery and why it is important for graduate (and undergraduate) college students to understand why. I offer suggestions that would have been helpful for me, but more importantly, suggestions to make people more effective in the world of counseling. Finally, there just had to be some final thoughts in the book about my love for all that is heavy in music, including some favorites, and the physical health aspect in recovery, which is vital in sustaining my recovery. How important is holistic health? It is a great way to accentuate your recovery, sustain your recovery, and give yourself the healing powers of self-care. For any person in recovery that is looking at becoming an addictions counselor, this book might be a good read to start your journey. Buckle up!!

PART I

Growing Up, the Rise of Addiction and the Denial of My Role as a Human

My early childhood was somewhat normal; I grew up fishing, playing sports, going to school, and doing "boy stuff." The years up to my adolescence were mostly good years, as my parents were pretty loving early on, and my younger brother Ed and I were the recipients of a lot of positive family support. There were holiday trips to my grandparents' house and yearly trips to French Lake in Faribault, where I would swim, fish, explore, and just have a great time. After my parents both passed away in early 2021, I was able to capture most of the pictures that my mother stored away, and they confirmed these thoughts on my childhood upbringing. We appear to be a happy family that took vacations, went to church, had a nice home, and had all of our needs met. My parents were both teachers, and they were both loving and kind. My father stayed that way his entire life, but he suffered from multiple sclerosis, which restricted his ability to move around, necessitating an assisted living facility. My mother, on the other hand, changed when I got older and started high school; she started to drift into making bad choices and horrible family decisions. When I officially became a teenager, something just changed in my mother. Her mental health became a big issue, and this led to some strict rules, punitive sanctions, and the inflicting of harm.

There were plenty of warning signs leading up to my first "drunk." Parenting really can affect some of the decisions children make in life. I am not going to blame anyone for my choice to drink and do drugs, as I earned it all through my actions. However, the authoritarian home in which I spent my adolescence was not conducive to love. My mother's parenting skills vacillated back and forth between authoritarian (when she was home) to neglectful (when she was home and away). Some of the first memories that

I have were the times when my parents would drop me off at my grand-mother's house and leave me there for weeks. I loved my grandma more than anything, and I didn't mind going there at all. However, what I call the "summer dump-off" happened for years. As I grew older, my mother was never home, and this was due to her "double life" as a cheater/adulterer. She was the epitome of selfishness. When she was home, she controlled my comings and goings, keeping me away from friends and girlfriends. She was overbearing, bound, and determined not to allow me to have any fun during my teenage years, despite the fact that I was basically playing sports, going to school, doing chores, etc. I wasn't in any trouble yet, but she punished me for being a normal kid. There were no dates, no prom, no senior class trip, and certainly no fun. I was basically on adolescent house arrest, and this fostered resentment and hatred. My father was a good man, hampered more and more by his disease. I had my father as a classroom teacher. My mother taught fifteen miles away. My dad's daily schedule was to teach and then come home and smoke two packs of Pall Malls while watching television with my brother. He lacked the assertiveness to stand up to my mother when she would invent new ways to ground me and prob-ably felt like his disease prohibited him from saying anything. My mother would get home after dark and fall asleep correcting spelling tests. She was in charge of this household, even though she was running around cheating on my father and was never home. My younger brother gravitated toward my father, and they were inseparable after school; watching television, eat-ing together, reading the paper, and being good pals. I loathed being idle, so I was always doing something. I would get home from sports practice and hole up in the basement, keeping to myself, as I was not given much of a chance to do anything else. I vividly remember holding out my left hand and throwing a tennis ball off the concrete walls of the basement, over and over again until I did not have to move my left hand to catch the ball. The repetition turned me into a very good catcher on the high school baseball team, and eventually won me a partial scholarship to play college baseball at the University of Northern Iowa. I also loved to play football in the fall and basketball in the winter. I would chip ice off the driveway for hours just so I could shoot hoops in sub-zero temps. I played sports twelve months out of the year and stayed away from the family as much as possible. I was not allowed much liberty and found solace in sports, a Stratomatic baseball game, and music. They kept me company, and I kept baseball statistics with the "spinner" game, which led to my love of numbers. I was not connected with the social part of my teenage years and I learned to be independent in order to amuse myself to the best of my ability. This is where my love of music grew, and I began to admire the "outcasts" of society, which is much of what bands like Black Sabbath, Iron Maiden, and the Misfits were singing about. It is interesting how I played sports all year long but did not spend my time with any jocks; instead, preferring the company of the school outcasts. My mother did not want me to date. She did not want me to be a teenager. She made me get a job my senior year, and I found one at a fast-food restaurant twenty miles away. My schedule became ridiculous, and this is where my resentment turned to bitterness and hatred. I would work from 8:00 pm to 3:00 am four nights per week, which messed up my sleep, my grades, and my senior season of baseball. I would get home at 3:30 am and have to get up for school at 7:00 am By the time I was ready to play baseball, I was absolutely exhausted. College coaches would come down to watch me play, and I would attempt to put on a show. I could not be on my "A" game, however, and I seethed inside. She was in control, which is what she must have wanted. She threw away all my letters from college baseball coaches, who were recruiting me to come to their schools and play. She also threw away my father's scrapbook, which was filled with sports clippings; I loved to go through it and read about him.

I do not know what happened to turn my mother into such a jealous, overbearing human, but I had just had enough. I made it until I graduated, and then, I was out of there. Good riddance to the controlling, emotionally abusive parent and to the other parent, who sat there and allowed it to happen. I understand how childhood experiences can affect what happens in adulthood, as hatred festers long after one leaves home—at least in my case. These are called adverse childhood experiences. My "innocent" alcohol use in 1986 progressed over the years and led me to dark and wretched places. The "taking of the soul" is not a quick process, as it happens insidiously, slowly, over time, so that everyone who watches the train wreck can see the progression but you. This slow decay is my descent into insanity.

First Drunk and The Seed was Planted

The first time I achieved "intoxication" was when I was seventeen years old, a late bloomer for a future alcoholic and drug addict. We had just won our first football game of my senior year, beating Rushford fourteen to eight. I was the QB/RB of the team and really thought I was a big deal. I went to a party, had too many beers, and vividly remember an old alum from Chatfield High School saying to me, "You are not going to be able to get away with drinking like this and also play quality football." I told him boldly, "I WILL drink like this AND be the best football player I can be." I was dropped off at my doorstep later that evening, passed out, and found by my parents at two o'clock in the morning with a quick doorbell ring and run. Four weeks later, I hurt my knee and missed the rest of the football season. Although I did not know it at the time, alcohol and drugs would eventually nudge out all my hobbies and passions and take center stage in my life. The rest of my senior year had some brief drinking stints, but I had little opportunity to drink, until I graduated.

The day I graduated high school, I grabbed a ride with some friends and moved away from home, running from the emotional abuse, the threat of rent, and the negativity that permeated that household. God, it was miserable there. If I was going to pay rent, it was not going to be under authoritarian rule, where I was being degraded and forced to stay at home while she went out and cheated on my father. I moved to St. Charles and found a place to live for eighty-five dollars per month. It was just an attic, but it was enough for me. I had a great summer, as I played the best baseball I have ever played, hitting almost .450, which transitioned me perfectly into fall baseball at UNI. I also started drinking a lot, as the place where I was renting was owned by the Swenson's, a family that "worked hard, played hard," which included Don, Greg, and Rick. Greg and Rick were Don's two sons, and Greg worked at Schott Distributing, peddling alcohol to bars and liquor stores. Don was a truck driver who enjoyed an adult beverage or two, and there was beer available all the time. Don had to drink his beer warm and hid it under his bed, as if it was in the fridge, we would drink it all. They were fun guys, and Greg and Rick were several years older than me and took me under their wing. I felt like I was part of a family, and it was a great summer with no consequences. Don was great to me, killing bats in my room and taping them to brooms with messages like, "Never fear, Underdog is here." They were just a friendly family with good humor, and we had some great times. We also partied heartily every weekend, with no letup at all. I drank to get drunk, plain and simple. I started to build up a tolerance and would drink until 4:00 am every Friday and Saturday. There were no bad times yet, and no negative consequences. I just remember this summer as a time of baseball, happiness, and a lot of laughs. I met my friend Mark in the summer of 1986, and he was heading for the Marines around the same time I was leaving for UNI. In the last month of summer, he would come and pick me up in the morning, and we would go on booze cruises all day long, resulting in daily intoxication and daily chaos. Mark would drink and drive, and we had some crazy days. We were really living on the edge of life and death, as we would drink a couple of cases of beer each day and hit the back roads. Looking back at this today, this was the time when I began to cross the invisible threshold from abuse to dependence. It was also the time when I became addicted to "high risk-taking behavior." This is an addiction all its own. I left for UNI in August of 1986 with the beginnings of an alcohol problem, a fresh start, and no idea what was going to happen next.

The College Train Wreck AKA the Shit Show

I wanted to get as far away from home as I could, so I decided to start my college years at UNI in Cedar Falls, Iowa. I was going there to play baseball, as I had carved out a nice high school sports career, with baseball and football being the two sports I loved with a passion. The two years in Iowa were both fun and somewhat useless at the same time. Being away from home and not having to deal with my immediate family was invigorating, but the years had created such hatred in my heart that alcohol became a way to forget that craziness. I lived in "Gold Falls" apartments, and the "off-campus" apartment complex housed football players, basketball players, wrestlers, and of course, the baseball team. It took some getting used to, but I took to the college and made friends fast. The apartment complex was just a perfect storm of unchecked male libido. Adding alcohol to that equation made for a breeding ground for the makings of a severe substance use disorder. I drank in earnest and hung out with ballplayers much older than myself, which put me in nonstop drinking situations. This didn't start immediately, however, and I maintained a 2.85 fall GPA while playing fall baseball. The spring was when my grades started to slowly sag, and I told myself it was because of the baseball season, but really, it was because I had found a core group of friends that loved to party on weekends. I was given a "redshirt" season but was allowed to play with the freshmen when they played the junior colleges and also be the bullpen catcher when the "big" team went on road trips. This was something I looked forward to, as I felt like I was paying my dues for future years, and also because my main peer group was the seniors on the team. When the season ended, I returned home for part of the summer, but of course, I brought my alcohol problem home with me. It travels well, no matter where you live. On June 27th 1987, I played a fastpitch softball game, drank ten beers on an empty stomach, and attempted to drive home. I fell asleep, and I flew off a very steep embankment in Troy, MN, plunging down hundreds of yards to the bottom. The radiator of the car was found in a tree. An older farmer heard the crash and called the police. They needed the Mayo One helicopter to get me out of there. The car looked like it had been hit by a tank. I needed well over a hundred stitches, and I vividly remember the EMT telling me how lucky I was to be alive as they cut off my shirt looking for damage. I also remember the police officer taking my blood to be tested for alcohol. My familiarity with the legal system was off and running, as the results showed a BAC of 0.10. This put my summer of playing sports on hold, and I got to UNI in August out of shape, rusty, and still healing. To make things even worse, the baseball coach who recruited me had left for another coaching job and had taken some of his best recruits with him—my friends. I did not like Gene Baker, the new coach. We did not hit it off well. I was not 100% healed from my injury from the DWI, and he must have found out that I decided to play fastpitch softball over the summer rather than baseball. What should have been my year to step up and be the full-time catcher became a year where I "platooned" with some converted outfielder and played about twenty-five games of the sixty-game schedule. Baseball was slowly starting to lose its luster, replaced by alcohol and drugs. I was pissed and resentful and I transferred after that year with a spring GPA of 0.87, and a cumulative of under 2.0. Alcohol had already gotten to the point where it was affecting my life. I had legal charges, handled my second year of college poorly, messed up my chance to play Division I college baseball for four years, and was now running from this school, back closer to home. My passions had switched from sports to partying. I had put myself into a hole and was forced to leave UNI, somewhat disgraced, but nothing compared to what was in store for me over the next twenty years.

Winona—
The Demon Seed Planted and Festering

The solution for me was to transfer to Winona State, where I knew a lot of people. I was going to play baseball, but had started to find the sport tedious, and I had lost a lot of the desire to play. Gary Raddatz was a scout for the Reds who also spent a lot of time in the fall watching Winona State baseball, and he knew me from scouting SE Minnesota in the past. He asked me what I did over the summer, and I told him I played fastpitch softball. He said, "What, don't you like baseball?" That comment stuck with me, as I really loved fastpitch softball. I played out the fall season, but when the coach told me I would have to take some make-up classes just to be eligible, I decided to get out of the game and focus on school and work. It was a surprisingly easy decision. I found a bartending job, was hired and started my first day of work on my twenty-first birthday. Putting a budding alcoholic behind a bar at the age of twenty-one was disastrous, and it laid the groundwork for the seedy underbelly of late nights, alcoholism, women, and drugs. The American Legion Club was my first bartending job, and the memories, although hazy, are still there. I must tell you that I met a great gal at UNI, and she was actually going to transfer with me to WSU. She was amazing, but I screwed that up badly when I started dating the Legion Club manager's daughter. She was a nice girl as well, but not Denise. She had minimal goals, and it was not a relationship I thought through very hard. When Denise and her father came to Winona to move all her stuff in, I told them both I was seeing someone else. It was a crushing blow to tell them, and although I was being honest, it tore me up. This is the selfishness of alcoholism at its worst. It just turns lives inside out. Working full-time as a bartender initiated a lot of alcohol-fueled decision-making, which became a huge downfall for me, including impulsive risk-taking. I started a series of "one-night stands" with single women, married women, old women—it just didn't matter. Some of these turned into longer relationships, but most of them were brief encounters. Some of the older Legion female members started to buy me things and invite me to Vikings games and other events. All I had to do was spend time with them in return. I don't know when exactly it happened but my morals and values began to lessen with my standards. This chapter at the American Legion ended after about eighteen months when I was terminated (this was to be a regular pattern for me over the years). They saw that I was giving free drinks to the day bartender, and they used this to get rid of me. However, by then, I was using my key to go there at all hours of the night, drinking and opening pull tabs. The Legion Board started to suspect things, as they would come in during the day, and the place would be a mess. I deserved to be let go; things were getting a little out of control. This led to another opportunity, as one of the Legion regulars was a bar owner, and he asked me if I wanted to work at his place. The "place" was called Ed's 500 Club, a no-nonsense type of bar where payroll checks would be cashed downstairs and dollar-twenty-five strong Bacardi Cokes would be slung out all night long. It was a "tough" neighborhood bar, and that is where I met my next roommate, who I lived with off and on for four years. This is where my drinking really escalated, and drug elements were added to the alcohol, including acid, methamphetamine, cocaine, weed, and mushrooms. The progression was immediate, but I did not really pay it much heed. However, my life was getting out of control fast. Our rented house became the spot for after bar parties, and we had some crazy nights/mornings. It is easy for me to sit here today and see how those years at Ed's 500 Club shaped my early adult years, as I can now see the trajectory my life was taking. When you are young, you think you are bullet-proof. My peer group really changed at this time, and my friends went from college students to "Winona lifers" that worked at factories and drank heavily. It was exactly what I wanted. My life was slowly becoming dominated by alcohol and drugs, especially on the weekends. It was not uncommon to have three or four "after bar" parties weekly, at my home after work because you could buy off-sale beer at Ed's. My roommate would bring a bunch of people back there, and when I would get home from working the bar, the place was already rocking. These nights began to just blend into each other—partying until the birds started singing (I hated that noise), going to school (or not going to school), and then getting ready for work, rinse, and repeat. During these years, patterns began to emerge, including the pattern of getting drunk and not caring about what I did or the consequences. I continued thinking I was "untouchable." Part of it was the crowd I was spending time with, and part of it was that I was starting to not care about anything. That is scary stuff. For example, I would pick up this crusty alcoholic at 8:00 am on Sunday for "church" across the river in Fountain City, Wisconsin. "Church" was the opening of The Cottonwood Bar, where we would go and get trashed. I had to pour the first two beers down his throat while he was still in bed because he was shaking so bad, and then he could put on his shoes, and we were off and running. I was entrenched in the drinking lifestyle, which was due to the decision to go and work at Ed's, and make that my priority. This was an education preparing me to move into the life of cocaine/meth/crime. I started to become enamored with this lifestyle and some of Ed's "regulars" became my friends, which meant I rarely had to struggle to find drugs. There was an attraction to spending time with "outlaws." I knew bikers who were peddling "crank," which was very pure methamphetamine. This tore me up to no end. I knew cocaine dealers and IV drug users who would come over to my place, put piles of coke on the table, and borrow my car for a couple of days. I remember taking an old sock that I was using as a dog toy and using it as a tourniquet to shoot up my friend George while I was tripping on acid. It is funny the things you remember about times like this. I saw myself becoming like these folks, and I started selling weed. I would buy an ounce each Friday and sell three quarters to receive the fourth for free. I would split this with my buddy Jay. My college grades suffered, and I ended up on the "seven-year plan," just like Bluto Blutarsky in *Animal House*. This went on ad nauseam, but by some miracle, I was able to make passing grades. I continued to plug along, getting my bachelor of science degree in teaching. I think my young age had something to do with my resilience, as well as my tolerance for alcohol. I just plodded along, putting minimal effort into school, but I was showing up for classes. I finally finished school and had the party of the year in Winona. My college graduation party was called the "Acid Alcohol (AA) Extravaganza," which consisted of a Wapatuli made out of $2000 worth of liquor, fruit, and mix; it filled a sixty-four-gallon garbage can. I had bought a sheet of acid, and I handed out one or two tabs for every interested person. It became a chaotic mess, which had simply become my "normal." I loved the danger of not knowing what was going to happen, so events like this became well-planned tickets to debauchery. I was simply "over the top" in my behaviors and actions. I was driving drunk, selling drugs, doing piles of hard drugs, and becoming well known as a partier. I was on the radar of the cops too. Once, they wanted me to become an informant, as they came to my home on a noise complaint, and I blew out a bong hit seconds before answering the door. They threatened me with charges, but I never heard from them again. I had gone from St. Charles to UNI to Winona, and I was now a full-blown alcoholic. Bartending put me around alcohol and around people that abused alcohol, and the old adage is true: You are who you spend most of your time with. Alcohol slowly became my center, and there was at least a little awareness of what was happening to my life.

When I look back at the Winona years today (1989-1994), those five years saw me use methamphetamine for the first time, bartend for the first time, start selling weed, and begin my addiction to drinking and driving (yes, it is an addiction), caught crabs (second time for that) and chlamydia (twice), and progressed to drinking daily. However, there were some accomplishments and lots of good times over these five years. I graduated with my bachelor's degree, I began coaching football, basketball, baseball, and softball at St. Stanislaus Catholic School, I went to Metallica twice (when they were good), and I saw the Twins win another World Series. I hadn't hit the bottom of the Jellinek Curve yet, but like a floating turd, I was eventually going to plummet to the bottom of the toilet.

I don't actually recollect how I got this job in 1992 (an ad in the paper, I think), but I spent about one year bartending in Caledonia, MN, at a supper club. I was very close to finishing college, as I had two classes to take, followed by a student teaching practicum. Caledonia was part of that equation, as I was hoping to pay for my summer classes out of pocket. Welcome to the Crest Supper Club, Bud and Dewey's Sealcoating, and another chapter in another town with similar results. After driving from Winona to Caledonia for three months or so, I ran into some folks who had an apartment for rent downtown. It made a lot of sense, and I took it. The move was simple (I had nothing). I played a little amateur baseball, but as I said before, I lacked the passion, as it had been replaced by partying. I was twenty-four, and it did not take long to find out who sold the weed, where the alcoholics lived, and who was available for romantic encounters. I was the new single-guy in a small town, and I took full advantage of that.

I easily could have destroyed two marriages but felt nothing, really, as these women presented themselves to me with no qualms. However, it was not a good look for me, and eventually I had to move back to Winona, as people were talking, and husbands were stalking. The summer of 1992 was a fun one, with still little to no consequences, although there could have been some disastrous ones. In a small town, you don't go around wrecking marriages, but I was young and dumb. I "dated" two of my co-workers and a lonely woman whose rich husband would go away on week-long trips. This had ramifications, and I had to get the hell out of there before one of these men decided to come after me. I had two angry husbands call my house and tell me to "leave my wife alone!" I was a disgraceful presence in that town and moved back in with my old roommate in Winona.

Getting Out of Winona
and the Move to Rochester

I spent the winter/spring of 1993 student teaching in Rochester at Hawthorne Elementary in Rochester, where I worked with Mrs. B and her sixth-grade class. I was able to stay with my parents in Rochester during the week and drove back to Winona on Friday to party with my roommate and the "boys." Mrs. B and I had a strange relationship, and although I was there every morning and I did a good job, I never felt comfortable in her classroom. She would watch me teach my lessons and take notes for the entire time, being overly critical. She did not give me many compliments. It did not appear like she wanted to have a student teacher, and I cannot really blame it on the alcohol, as the only day I was really hurting was on several Mondays. I don't know if she smelled alcohol on my breath on some of those Monday mornings, but she did not give me a glowing report at the end of my experience (my University Supervisor did). I was very resentful of her for this. This experience was my resume at this point, and it didn't help that I already had a DWI on my record. I had nothing on my resume that made me stand out, which hindered the opportunity to even get an interview. I remember going to a job fair where teachers were being recruited for states like Texas. I drove to the fair and could not even get an interview. I was frustrated but I was also not putting in anything better than a "C" effort. After graduating from college in May 1993, I wallowed around Winona for about one year, sending out some applications and working at Canamer International. I worked 6:00 pm to 6:00 am the entire summer and fall of 1993, making huge tarps to send to Iran to put on rock piles. We had a monster order for about 200 of these to be completed by the end of the year, and in one twelve-hour shift, we could make two, possibly three of them. It was a job, but nothing else. I worked eighty-four hours weekly for most of the summer. I learned to love "white crosses," which are basically truck stop speed, containing the ingredient ephedrine. I would eat ten or more of those nightly, which would make the shift fly by. Marijuana was smoked copiously at breaks, but there wasn't much time for any other drugs. I slept during the day and went to work my job when people were leaving theirs. The hours were not conducive to having a life but were perfect for a vampire. The only thing that was really memorable about working there was getting a bonus on New Year's Eve and spending the entire $600 on cocaine in one day. I was supposed to take a girl out to eat, and she found me wandering the "projects" at about seven, looking for more. She made me take her out to Finn and Sawyers and then to a bar, where I was snorting a line of coke off the back of the toilet at midnight. I was just a classy guy back then. Canamer was a job, but that was all, and I worked there until the summer of 1994. I made the decision to move to Rochester in the fall of that year because I was going to substitute teach in Rochester and try to "get my foot in the door" of the teaching profession. I was told that a male elementary teacher would be in high demand, but I needed to get some experience and meet some teachers. I packed my meager belongings to move in September of 1994, but my alcoholism got in the way again as I procured a DWI on the last leg of moving my stuff to Rochester. I was going back to Winona to spend the night at my friend's and then bring the last few items to Rochester the next day. I was pulled over for speeding coming into Winona. My blood alcohol level was 0.11, and I was charged with my second DWI. During the ride to the police station, I was given the opportunity to be handcuffed in front, and I was able to get my wallet out of my pocket and ingest the potent chunk of weed I had hidden in there for my friend and me to smoke. It was wrapped in cellophane, and I had to really work hard to swallow it. I "passed" that three days later, and it was still intact, although the cellophane had started to unravel. I hit the weed with a blow dryer and smoked it—the true definition of "shit weed." This was my initiation to Rochester in 1994. I now had two DWIs on my record, and my portfolio was beginning to look very unappealing to prospective employers. I remember that first year of substitute teaching well because I took jobs at any school where there were openings. I think I taught about eighty percent of the school days and was starting to get to know the local teachers. I really was getting my foot in the door. I was living with my parents at the time and was somewhat protected from myself (I needed it). After getting established in Rochester, I moved out and found my own apartment. Soon after that, something happened in the fall of my second year of substitute teaching, and I lost the ability to substitute teach. A student got in trouble and told on me, stating that we were talking about marijuana in class (we were). The student went home and told his parents, and I was out as a substitute teacher. Due to that boundary issue and transgression, I needed to find work. I didn't have my driver's license due to my DWI in 1994, so I found more menial work as a janitor and at Textile Care. I felt my options were dry, which is why I chose to go back to menial work akin to Canamer in Winona. I had a bachelor's degree and was hanging clothes for eight hours and then cleaning the same building for four hours. I was barely making ends meet, however, which did curtail my drinking to some extent. I was also riding a bicycle at that time, so if I wanted beer I had to stash it in my backpack. These jobs lasted about six months, and then I made the decision to go back to bartending. I restarted this process in the fall of 1995, starting at King's Krossing, and I also bartended at Sandy Point Supper Club, Colonial Lanes, Mr. Bowser's, and Recreational Lanes (now called Bowlocity). These three years of bartending saw me slow down on substitute teaching and go into full-time drink slinging, although I did coach ninth-grade boys' basketball at Rochester Lourdes and was the tenth-grade football coach at Plainview High School. This Lourdes coaching gig was a good one for me, as it probably slowed down the progression of my alcoholism. I applied for the job and had two good interviews before getting hired in 1994. I had two great teams and one good team, and of course, being an alcoholic, I took way too much credit for coaching ball players who had already taken the sport seriously for years. Our record the first year was thirty-two and three, followed by twenty-nine and six, and then twenty and eleven. The parents of the kids at this private Catholic school were clamoring for me to take over the varsity job, and this also went to my head. Those three years there were a blast, and other than a few very minor scrapes with the head coach, I thought I did a wonderful job. I was not retained after my third year and found out through a parent of one of the boys I coached, who spilled the news to me at a grocery store. I was just hired to help coach the "B" squad football team at Lourdes, but I decided that this news was enough to say, "To hell with Lourdes," and I turned it down. I was hurt, but I know I showed up for weekend tournaments with alcohol on my breath, and people smelled it. I also know they wanted a teacher to take this job, and they found one. This one stung, and it increased my drinking once again, as well as my drug use.

King's Krossing was akin to Ed's 500 Club, and I quickly embraced the drug lifestyle again. At King's, I worked Friday during the day and then Sunday and Monday nights. My shifts at the Bowling Alley were Friday and Saturday nights, so I only worked four days, but I worked great tipping shifts. I made good money, got free food from places where I worked, and started drinking and doing drugs in large amounts. My tip jar at King's was usually full of money AND different drugs, including weed, shrooms, powdery substances (either meth or cocaine), and acid. I started seeing a married (but separated) woman who was older but treated me very well. I remember getting home from a long shift bartending, throwing all my tips on the floor, letting her count them, and smoking a big joint. We would get high, drink, and have a lot of fun. It was awesome, and she was a great partner. However, my life once again began to slowly unravel as the progression of my addiction gained speed, and methamphetamine made another appearance in my life. I messed up again and started dating a young, attractive, budding drug addict named Melissa, discarding Vicky like she was a bag of garbage. Melissa and I moved in together in 1997. She liked to drink and smoke pot, and we had a good relationship for one year, but it just fizzled. She started going out with her girlfriends all night, and I got jealous and started to resent this behavior. We broke up around the time I was hired as a bar manager. My bartending jobs were enough to make ends meet, but one day I received a call from an old friend from St. Charles, who stated they were looking for a bar manager at the Moose Lodge in St. Charles. I thought it was a decent opportunity to make extra money and have a job with a tiny bit of prestige. My alcoholism was a big problem, but I still thought this was going to be a successful endeavor. It simply became another chapter involving embarrassment and disgrace.

I moved into the country and rented a trailer in the middle of nowhere. Actually, it was about ten miles from St. Charles and about five miles from Chatfield in a small "hamlet" called Troy. The trailer was about two miles from my car accident in 1987. I took the Moose Lodge job and started in August of 1998. I had nothing to lose, as I was not coaching anymore and had no reason to remain in Rochester. I knew plenty of people who lived in St. Charles that were members of the Moose Lodge. The fall went great, and I started to fill the bar with old members and some new members. I was playing fastpitch softball for a St. Charles team, and the Moose Lodge sponsored us, adding to our membership, and bringing a younger element into the Lodge. A lot happened over the eighteen months I worked at the "Moose." I was handed the administration job, which came with more responsibility. The newness of this opportunity was refreshing, and I started to feel a little better about myself. However, being around alcohol all day was a recipe for disaster. The bar was entirely mine, and I vividly remember tapping myself a Foster's Lager when I got there in the late morning before doing anything else. I lived by myself, and there was no accountability, so with that, all of what happened next was just inevitable. I was drinking on a Saturday night, and I received my third DWI in the early summer of 1999. I was over the bridge in Wisconsin with two peers on my fastpitch team at 2:00 am, being somewhere I had no business being. On the drive home, a cop drove past me, and he stated I was in the wrong lane and almost killed him. I do not doubt I was partially in the other lane. I had messed up again. This was the first time I had to actually do jail time, as it was my third overall DWI. There was nothing I could do about it and I was given thirty days in jail. I started my jail stint in the late summer and I was given work release privileges. Melissa felt sorry for me and would come and pick me up at 2:00 pm and then drive me back to the jail by 2:00 am. I was given good time, so this should have been a twenty-day sentence, which is no big deal. I managed to mess this up royally and about lost my job because of it. I drank throughout my work release jail sentence but would quit about 8:00 pm, six hours before I was to report back to the jail. On my last night, they joked about giving me a breathalyzer, but this was no joke. I blew a 0.10, and lost my ten days of good time. I had to sit in jail for ten more days without work release privileges. This put a strain on my job and some of the people who were stepping in for me in my absence. I was almost fired and had to sign a "no use contract," which made me get very sneaky about my drinking. I also had to attend outpatient treatment, which I did in Rochester. I drank my way through that treatment program, meeting some good guys who would come to the Moose Lodge and drink with me on Sundays for football games.

I met "Debbie" in 1999 at a St. Charles class reunion at Good Sport, and we hit it off. She told me the first night we met that she was an alcoholic, and I said, "good." What followed was an eight-year relationship that could best be described as chaotic and filled with drinking and drugs. As I met a new group of people in St. Charles, and more of my fast-pitch softball teammates were coming in to drink, I started to have after-bar parties at the Lodge. They quickly progressed to weekly endeavors and the bar was packed. We had to have people park a couple of blocks away, as cops would drive by and wonder what was going on as the lights were on. These would last until 4:00 or 5:00 in the morning on Friday and Saturday nights. Eventually, board members found out and addressed it in a board meeting with me. There was a Saturday morning pool tournament, and I had left the place an absolute mess Friday night. My undoing at the Lodge was becoming apparent. People were not paying for drinks, and I was slinging a lot of them for free. I had scheduled a vacation to Mexico with a group of people from February twelfth to the twentieth, and prior to leaving St. Charles, all thirty-five of us assembled at the Moose Lodge on a Friday afternoon. We had drinks, figured out who was going in what car and left for Minneapolis to stay overnight, and then hit the airport. I had not been on a vacation since 1993, when I drove to Vermont to drop a friend off. This Mexico vacation was a disaster, as alcohol, cocaine, and marijuana were plentiful. I turned my ankle the first day there, and it became very swollen. I was so intoxicated I did not even feel it until the fifth day. I met some other Minnesotans, and we golfed, drank, and had a crazy, wild time. I was ready to go back long before the vacation was over. We got back on a Saturday, and when I walked into the Moose Lodge to get my keys, an eerie quiet fell in the bar. I sensed something was amiss, but I was so tired that I just grabbed my keys and went home. When I was going through my mail, there was a letter from the Moose Lodge, terminating me and setting up a February twenty-first meeting to hand in keys, etc. They fired me while I was on vacation. Yes, I deserved it, but it created another resentment. These resentments I carried through my twenty-two years of drinking could have easily killed me, and certainly elevated my levels of stress and anger. When I showed up the next morning to get my last check and hear them out, they chastised me like I was a ten-year old that was late for school. "You partied at the bar after hours; you were not doing your job, you have a drinking problem, you are disrespectful, blah, blah, blah." They were right on all counts, and I don't blame them one bit for doing what they did. I came back from Mexico penniless and lost my job on top of it. It is funny how life works when you are an alcoholic. You truly live one day at a time as an addict, just like people do in recovery. I never thought ahead, never thought I would lose my job while on vacation, and never thought of the consequences. I just barreled forward with no clue, trying to dominate everything in my sight. This is the story of my addiction. I would be just moving along, drinking, drugging, not planning, not thinking of anything, and then BAM. . .DWI, loss of a job, time in jail, etc. Everything would come crashing down, and I would be left shaking my head, going, "What the hell just happened?" It was now 2000, and alcohol and drugs had been dominating me for years; the insanity of doing the same thing over and over again and expecting different results. Sadly, I still had seven years of beatings left to take, and these beatings eventually broke me.

I started applying for jobs, and in what has been a common theme in my hazy years of addiction, I have no idea why I applied at the Rochester Golf and Country Club, other than they must have been looking for a bartender. I had about eleven years of bartending experience and was able to draw on that to secure this job. I started in approximately March of 2000. This was a new experience for me, as I had worked at some pretty "rough and tumble" bars such as Ed's 500 Club and King's Krossing. This place was home to the "elite" of Rochester, as far as status and money go. Radio station owners, surgeons and doctors at the Mayo Clinic, and construction conglomerates all had memberships there, not to mention the golfers I met in this bunch. For the most part, I got along well with all of them. I was serving them drinks, and on the weekends, I was serving their wives drinks. I got to see some of them in the throes of intoxication, which humanized them to me. I met some "heavy hitters" who would tip me outrageous sums to run them drinks on Friday afternoons. They would call on me while they were on various holes on the golf course. I would make them strong margaritas and jump on a golf cart and bring them out to them. When the night was over and their families had eaten, members would leave hundred-dollar bills on the tables when they left. I forged a relationship with several of the members and eventually, I was invited to bartend their personal and professional Christmas parties at their homes. I saw alcoholism amongst the rich, and it was thrilling to be able to bartend at these parties. I worked five of them all together. However, it was Labor Day weekend in

2000 that I will forever remember about that year, as I picked up my fourth DWI on a Saturday night. This DWI sticks out because I was not working on a Saturday night, which was rare. I was drinking at my favorite watering hole, the North Star Bar, and, as is usually the case, I ran into someone who had drugs. He had just "whipped up a batch" of methamphetamine. I preferred cocaine but methamphetamine worked as well. He invited me to his place, where he was drying it. He was just finishing up and gave me a quarter gram. It was a good batch!! I decided to try to get home that night and waited at a friend's house until about 2:00 am because I knew I was drunk. I was supposed to be getting onto a bus at 8:00 am to go to the Vikings' home opener against Chicago. I felt fine taking off, but driving through small towns at 2:00 am is asking for trouble, and I was pulled over for allegedly taking a left turn too sharply. I passed the field sobriety tests, but he gave me the test and I blew yellow which finally turned red. It was a 0.11 BAC. This was the only time I asked the officer for a break, telling him I waited at a friend's house for five hours until I felt safe to drive. He wasn't having it, and I was booked and held in jail for the rest of Labor Day weekend. This was DWI number four, and the consequences were steadily increasing. I was given ninety days in jail, but I could do half on Electronic Home Monitoring. I was able to keep my job at the Country Club, but I had to tell them. I did the forty-five days on EHM at my parent's house, so I could bike to work, as I obviously lost my license (and my car). Things had soured at the Country Club, and I was tired of it. The golf season was over, and things had slowed down. My hours were cut, but I was able to bartend at some Christmas parties at the Club. I was also asked to bartend at some members' houses for Christmas parties and this is how I lost my job. I had bartended four of them and had an opportunity to make it five. However, it was on a night I worked (Friday night). I called in sick so I could bartend for a doctor's Christmas party for friends. I knew this one was going to be fun, as I had already bartended at his place when he threw a Christmas party for his co-workers/colleagues. He paid me $400, which was so much more than I would get for working at the club on a winter Friday night with few customers. Well, they found out, and when I showed up the next shift, they sent me packing. However, due to getting fired from job after job, I started to figure out backup plans. I had met a man who managed Digger's Bar and Grill in Kasson one day at work, as he was a golfing guest of a

Country Club member. I hung onto his phone number, and once I was jettisoned out of the club, I gave him a call and had an interview. I was hired and started less than one week later. This brings me to the year of chaos, with equal parts insanity and nightmares. Both were offered up liberally. I will never forget this year and the craziness involved as I literally put my life (and others) in my hands daily. I lost all semblance of caring for anyone else, especially myself, and went on a one-year blackout, courtesy of alcohol and drugs, of course. It was insane, and to top it off, I was on probation for four lifetime DWIs. I cared not one bit.

Digger's Bar and Grill was located in Kasson, MN, and it was about forty-five miles from my home in rural Chatfield. I was now operating without a driver's license, so I had to be careful, which included strapping up the seat belt and not speeding. I had an old Delta 88 that I drove for about half the year, and then I was able to start driving my grandmother's Buick after she passed away. To describe Digger's would be simple: Close enough to Rochester to attract that crowd, located right next to a motel that attracted a crowd, good food to attract a crowd, right off Highway 14 to attract people, and a karaoke machine to attract wannabe singers. I started in January as a part-time bartender, working weekends (when they needed two bartenders). I had become a good bartender, as I had the gift of gab, could talk sports and could sling drinks with the best of them (lots of practice). I believe I started to threaten the full-time bartender a little, and he was getting burnt out. He was fired one night for his attitude, and I took his hours, so I was working Monday, Tuesday, Thursday, Friday, and Saturday nights. This set the stage for my debauchery, and I continued to pay the price with my life (or what resembled a life).

Every time I moved to a new place or worked in a new town or city, it was easy for me to meet people, thanks to the bartending trade. This was no different. I met lots of new people and was well-liked by my co-workers. This was by far my favorite bartending job due to my co-workers, the amount of tip money I made, and the fact that it did not take me long to discover that I was pretty much in charge of the place five nights per week. Mondays, Tuesdays, and Thursdays were good tipping nights, but Fridays and Saturdays were ridiculously busy. I got a second bartender at 8:00 pm both nights, so I was on my own from 5:00 pm to 8:00 pm. I made some decent money those three hours but from 8:00 pm to 1:00 am the place was packed. Management brought in two professionals who did the karaoke weekend, and as this was a newer fad, people just ate it up. I would make $200 each night after dividing up the tips, and that was consistent. I had money, lived by myself in the country, and drank every day. I went to many concerts that year, including Rammstein, Slipknot, Tool, Pantera, Machine Head, Slayer, Morbid Angel, and System of a Down. It was a wonder I did not pick up my fifth DWI while I worked there. However, the craziness and legal ramifications affected me, nonetheless. I had romantic endeavors left and right and did not care with who. I was still technically dating my girlfriend, but she moved to St. Paul, so "out of sight, out of mind." I thought I was untouchable, as I would leave the bar at 2:00 am with a twelve-pack and a bottle in my hand. There would be cops in the parking lot that would wave to me and wish me a good night. They called me "Rick" because I had insurance in his name. I did not have a driver's license, had racked up four DWIs, was intoxicated, and I was ready to drive forty-five miles home. The cops just nodded at me and let me go on my way. I felt like I could do anything, as in ten feet tall and bulletproof, and I would bask in the temporary glow of "fucking the system." I wasn't braindead enough to think this was going to last forever, but until I was caught, I was going to have a merry good time. As I said previously, I really didn't care anymore about anything. I was just living the alcoholic bartender dream. I was a bloated 230 pounds, was on probation in Olmsted County, and was lying my teeth off to my probation agent every month. Little did I know that she was giving me chances to come clean and kept a tally of my lies. She was also giving me witnessed urine tests, and I had three in a row that were positive for a different substance every time: Marijuana, cocaine, and methamphetamine. I was digging myself a hole and lacked care and awareness. The fun could never last, and to be honest, as I sit here and type this, it lasted longer than it should have. My routine was as follows: Worked on Monday, Tuesday, Thursday, Friday, and Saturday—would drink and drive every night after work. I would get drunk on Monday, drunk on Tuesday (I was off Wednesday, but drunk), drunk on Thursday, drunk Friday, drunk Saturday, and drunk Sunday (you get the point). I started work at 5:00 pm and would usually pour my first Captain & Coke after the waitress ordered one, as then I could pour two. I had four to five Captains in the first several hours per workday and then switched to Grey Goose Vodka and orange energy drink (in a twenty-two-ounce soda glass). I would drink six of those and then it would be time to close the bar. While I was closing the bar I would drink two beers, so by the time I was heading to my car, I had roughly twenty drinks in me. Now on Friday and Saturday nights, I would take home a twelve-pack and/or a Styrofoam glass filled with vodka and drink and drive on the way home. I would stop at my friend's house to pee and throw empty bottles in his driveway. The law of averages allows this type of behavior for a certain amount of time, and then something happens to get tripped up. In this case, it was my probation officer, but it could have been another DWI, hitting a deer, killing someone, killing myself. I am ashamed to say that I woke up multiple times to look outside and see if my car was in the driveway (the car I should not have been driving because I did not have a license). Some readers that don't understand the progression of alcoholism may lose any semblance of empathy for me at this point, as the selfishness was over the top, and I had no care for myself or others. To be blunt, this is how addiction works. When you are in the midst of it, you will do things that are shameful and embarrassing. There is still some shame in how I acted during those last years of drinking, but I want the reader to know how low life had gotten.

I would attend my PO appointments prior to going to work, so we had them scheduled for about 3:30 pm. I would park about six blocks from the government center, as I did not have a driver's license, and I needed a safe place for my car if I was going to be put in jail on a probation violation. This happened often (I was booked into Olmsted County alone ten times). I would go in and see her monthly and would sweat out the entire day, as a urine screen could pick up any of the following drugs on a given day: Alcohol, marijuana, cocaine, and methamphetamine. When she started to give me these urine screens consistently, I was not able to take a clean one. My first one was positive for marijuana, the second one for cocaine, and the third one for methamphetamine. There was alcohol in all of them. I would lie and lie and lie, but this all came to a head one day in the fall of 2001. I had a regularly scheduled appointment with "Linda," and when I got into her office, she started asking me questions. "Are you still working at The AmericInn?" This motel was right next to the bar, and I gave the motel manager free drinks if she or one of her employees would run and grab me if probation ever called looking for me. I would then run over there and pick up the phone. She had no problem doing this, as I would also stay at the motel sometimes and sleep with her. Anyway, I answered that question, "Yes." The next question was, "Are you still attending outpatient treatment/aftercare at FC?" I hadn't been going there for six months, and I can't even remember how long I attended FC that time. However, I said, "Yes." The next question was, "Are you getting rides to work?" "Yes," I stated. "Are you remaining sober?" "Yes, Linda." Are you attending AA meetings?" "Yes." This "Q & A" went on for some time, and she finally stated to me, "Do you realize you just lied to me in every answer you gave me?" For the first time in two years, I looked at her and told her the truth. "Yes." They brought up the turnkeys, and I was taken down the elevator to booking and jail. This was to become a common occurrence for the next several years, as I previously mentioned (I was given the booking photos of those "experiences" in 2017, and eight photos are displayed in this book). This time, Linda decided to execute my sentence, and I ended up getting a year in jail. I lost my job at Digger's, and my time in jail increased. In the interim, I ended up finding a job at the Preston B&B as a cook. This was an ok job, but of course, there were no tips and no easy access to alcohol. I was to start my jail sentence in May 2002, and I don't know how I managed this, but I ended up getting back on the Rochester Sub Finder and got a teaching job at John Adams Middle School that ran through May. I also ended up finding a job at the Stewartville Golf Course, so I could do work release when jail started. This meant I could leave the jail during the day and go to work, but I had to pay the jail one-hundred-and forty-dollars per week for the privilege. It was worth it. I was figuring things out again. This was my pattern, as I would put myself in a hole and then bust my ass to find employment and start to dig my way out.

I turned myself in for my jail stint the Tuesday after Memorial Day weekend in 2002 and started my bit. I was hoping for eight months with good time. I enjoyed working at the golf course, and I had my neighbors looking after my dog. I would leave work on Saturdays and run home to check my mail and see my dog. I would then go back to jail. I was driving without a license, so I would park by Deb's house (my girlfriend, remember her?). She moved back to Rochester in the interim and was living in an efficiency. We were still together, as much as two tragic alcoholics can be together. However, I was still drinking during my work shifts. I would get back to the work release facility at about 1:30 am. I would have to buzz to get myself in. There was an African American jailer who would be working on many of those nights, and he liked to sleep on his shift. He would buzz me in, but wouldn't check me and he would just let me go to my room. I started to figure out his work patterns and I would drink heavy amounts of alcohol on the nights he was working. I would be buzzed in, go into the room to change, and be buzzed into the unit to go up to my cell. This was a great way to do time, I thought. Getting drunk and then going to jail to sleep, wake up, and wait until I was allowed to go back to work. However, you all know how this is going to end up, right? Deb tried to warn me about this when I was struggling to put my pants on one night. She said, "You are never going to get away with this, Tim." I didn't get caught that night, but two weeks later, I did. There was actually a turnkey there who was doing her job! She allowed me to go up to my cell, but about 30 minutes later, I heard someone's boots trudging up the stairs. I knew I was doomed once again. I blew numbers for alcohol and had to speak to the Director of the jail the next day. I lost my job, and worst yet, the main unit was full, so they sent me to Carver County in Chaska. No one knew I was there, and I began my rehabilitation in the place where they were holding the U.S. Open that year. I was in for a long summer and fall.

Carver County jail was not a good place. They were "hosting" inmates from other facilities and getting paid by the county of origin. I was put in the INS unit, where Hispanic folks were being held until deportation. Some had been in there for eighteen months. There were four guys to a room with no doors on the cells. It was a smelly, foul place to call home for five months. Guys didn't like shitting in front of the whole unit, so they would go into the showers and poop in there. They would then proceed to attempt to stomp it down through the grates in the drain. Eventually, this backfired, and they plugged up. Guys were sent into their cells for twenty-four-hour lockdowns on a recurrent weekly pattern. Fortunately, I had put in a "kite" for a kitchen worker. After spending about one month in there, I was able to get that kitchen job, which allowed me to have a cell of my own and get some purpose. I was down in the kitchen from 5:30 am to 6:30 pm Monday through Sunday, and I got one day off my sentence for each day worked. I only had to work from 5:30 am to 2:30 pm, but there was a radio down there, fresh laundry daily, and I just stayed as long as I could.

I served all three meals, prepped, did the dishes, and folded laundry. I also lost almost fifty pounds, as I began watching my diet down in the kitchen. I ate a strict carb diet of one meal per day, was not drinking (obviously), and did as much physical health stuff as I could. This included 500 push-ups nightly after working in the kitchen all day. I went into jail weighing over 230 pounds and came out of jail at less than 190 pounds. My time shrunk by almost one-hundred days, and I was released home on October 6th, 2002—a one-year sentence was whittled down to about 140 days, with good time and work privileges. Physically, this was the best I felt in years, as I had sustained my sobriety for almost six months, had dropped a lot of weight, had clarity, and had a lot of time to think about which direction my life was going to go in next. You would think that someone should have had enough at this point. I was off probation for the first time in three years, and I could have started rewriting my story at the age of thirty-four, which would have made a huge difference in my life. Alcoholism and addiction do not work that way, however. When you are not done, you are not done. There needs to be something greater than yourself to guide you in the right direction. I had put in the work to make the most out of my jail stint and had benefited from being in a controlled environment, basically in solitude. This is something that always stuck in the back of my head years before I was to be a counselor. It is easy to stay sober in a controlled environment, but if you are not getting any programming to build skills or prepare you for when you get out of this controlled environment, you will just revert back to your old ways. It is like putting the stylus back on the record album and having it move over the same grooves to play the same songs. If you desire change, you have to try something different (like a different album). I did not take advantage of this "gift" and reverted back to old ways fast.

I was released from jail on a Sunday morning, and my pasty self was picked up by my friend Will. The Twins were playing Oakland in game five of the divisional series, and we watched that at his place. I had him drop me off after the game (Twins won the series that day, which is why I remember that date so much) at Deb's place, and when I opened the fridge, it was loaded with vodka and Twisted Teas. My five months of forced sobriety were over. I started my self-destruction immediately, as we decided to go to a bar for Game One of the Twins/Angels AL Championship Series. We were riding bikes, and I got so intoxicated during the game I was kicked out. I jumped on my bike and fell off going down a hill, messing up my shoulder (I still have a nice calcium deposit on my shoulder blade). In the interim, my parents took all my possessions and threw them in their yard, as I did not go over there after being released. They were so put out by having my meager possessions there that they decided to toss them in their front yard. I moved in with my friend Will for two months, which was seven or eight miles out of town. I started riding a bike and began substitute teaching, as Will was sober, and it was good to be away from Rochester and the easy access to alcohol. After subbing for two months, I found a place in Rochester, and I also found a teaching job at Burr Oak School. Burr Oak was a Level IV E/BD behavioral setting for students who have been expelled from the Middle Schools and High Schools for anything from excess absences to bringing a knife to school to drug charges or possession. They were willing to take any warm body with a pulse to work there. I was that warm body. However, I was excited to be able to have my own classroom and my own students. This was an opportunity that could have opened the door for better opportunities, but alcohol and cocaine once again got in the way.

I began working at Burr Oak in December of 2002 and also began renting a home around this time as well. This was a nice home, and Debbie moved in with me. After my bicycle mishap, I did not drink a lot. I settled in and started to get back into the schools, deciding to leave bartending behind. Living with Will and substitute teaching gave me some structure, and I took advantage of that two-month period of time. I am grateful to Will and the opportunity he gave me during that time. Living with him was my version of staying at a halfway house.

Burr Oak was not an enjoyable place to work, but I already knew that. These students came from broken families, where poverty, drugs, and crime were center stage. However, I was excited to be using my college degree and to have my own classroom. Part of the stipulation of being hired there (and the next year as well) was that I re-enroll in school and start graduate courses in Special Education, as my degree was in Elementary Education. As long as I was working toward this master's degree, I would be hired on a year-by-year variance. Listen, no one wanted this job, as it was stressful, the kids were tough as nails, and we couldn't even get anyone to sub there. I had nothing to worry about as long as I was enrolled in courses. I started college in the spring of 2003. I was also hired at Barnes and Noble, which would be part of my summer plans, as I would need to stay busy, and I could make a little extra money. My schedule was brutal: I was taking two classes and had to drive (without a license) to Mankato twice per week. I had to be at my job around 6:30 am, and school was let out at 2:00 pm. Classes at Mankato State were at 5:00 pm, so I had basically an hour to eat, change clothes, and get on the road. I also worked about twenty-four hours per week at B&N. This set the table for me to have some serious structure, which limited my drinking. But as any good alcoholic will tell you, we will find a way. I had racked up four DWIs, mind you, and was driving without a license. In my distorted thinking, it sounded like a great idea to start pulling into the Janesville liquor store on Thursday nights on the way back from Mankato to buy booze. So...after a long day, starting at 5:00 am, I would start drinking at 8:30 pm and drive home. I was certainly not thinking of the long-term ramifications my next offense would give me (I never thought about that), and was certainly not thinking of my career or the goals I had set for myself. It was just part of my self-defeating pattern. If you are reading this and saying to yourself, "What in the world is he doing?" You are not alone. People who were close to me just shook their heads and had to walk away from me, as it was too painful to watch. Trust me; it has been painful to write as well.

Going into the summer of 2003, I found out that I was hired back for the full school year starting in 2003-2004. This school was not conducive to longevity, as the kids were tough to work with, and the burnout rate was high. I was grateful for this opportunity, which included continuing in school, and working at Barnes and Noble. I had structure and some semblance of normalcy, but like most other things in my life during this time, I took it for granted. My life was as good as it could get for this alcoholic, I thought. Looking at this today is another example of me "settling," as alcohol was the priority, and everything else falls under that category. I was one small mishap away from another disaster.

I began my school year in August of 2003, and things felt good. I was teaching from the beginning of the year, so there was some normalcy to the job. I received a caseload of clients, which were damaged teenagers, of course. I was damaged myself, which is why I think they looked at me differently than the other teachers. They could sense I was one of them, as they grew up with alcoholic parents and broken homes. We were trained in crisis intervention, which included restraining students if they posed a risk to themselves or others. It was a tough facility to teach at, and certainly, the stress of the job contributed to my alcoholism. However, by then, I was already in deep, so I certainly didn't need any excuses. I attempted to control my drinking by picking and choosing my spots. I tried hard!!! Monday was work and "Whistle Binkies" day. I would get off work at 3:00 and go drink there. Once good and drunk, I would order food and go home. Tuesday was a Barnes and Noble evening. Wednesday and Thursday were "drive to college" days, and Thursdays I imbibed on the way home from Mankato. Friday night, I tried to take it easy, as Saturday. I worked a full day shift at Barnes and Noble. When I got off work at 5:30 pm, it was straight to McCormick's bar, where I would drink two jelly jars of Long Island Iced Tea and then go to the liquor store. I would drink at home and listen to GG Allin, (another master of self-destruction to which I could relate), then hit the North Star Bar on Saturday to listen to some metal and look for the after-bar parties. I would find cocaine there to entice people to come with me to the party. I was now living by myself, and parties were the norm on a Saturday night. Sunday, I would recover and do some main-tenance drinking. My teaching job suffered. I was not on top of my game there, and colleagues were starting to notice this. People smelled alcohol on my breath when we were doing restraints. Colleagues started making comments like, "my mother was an alcoholic." I started crossing bound-aries with the mother of one of my students. She would buy me sports jerseys and put them under my car. We started an intimate relationship. I was already in a relationship, so chaos was inevitable. I "hung on" until the fateful days of April 30th to May 1st of 2004. This Friday night into Saturday morning is etched into my core to this day for multiple reasons, and it was the first time I had entertained thoughts of suicide.

I remember bits and pieces of that day, and one thing that sticks out is that I was at the bar Friday night, which was not normal. I normally worked a long Saturday day shift at Barnes and Noble, and I was sched-uled to work that next morning. I hated going in there with zero sleep and hung over. Anyway, I ended up at the North Star Friday night, got drunk, and was on the prowl for cocaine or crack. Some random guy stated he could help me out, and we ended up back at my place. When you are smoking crack and drinking, time gets away from you. It was about four in the morning when I decided I wanted him out. I had spent all my money on crack and had nothing to give him for a cab. He had no money......so I made the mistake of driving him home. Now, I had expired tags on my car (the license plate wasn't even the correct one), and I knew cops were on the prowl looking for drunk drivers at that time of the morning. However, I did it anyway. I did not make it far, and a cop started to follow me. I knew this was it. The tags would be seen, and that would be excuse enough to pull me over. I started to navigate my way back closer to my house, and the lights went on. I continued driving, upsetting my passenger. Finally, I pulled over about four blocks from my house and got out, and started running for home. I had locked the door when leaving, so I had to break into a basement window to get in. I sat in my room with the lights off and listened. About ten minutes later, I heard noises. They were at the house and started knocking at the door. I had pieces of mail in my car, left the car running, and stranded my passenger on the side of the road. There was no doubt they were going to find the house. Well, I was going to make the cops do their job, so I sat in there for what seemed like hours. Finally, they broke down the door and came into the bedroom with guns on me, screaming at me to "hit the floor." The city block was lit up like the 4th of July. One cop made a snide remark as I was led out the door in handcuffs, "He will never teach again." That haunted me for years and also gave me further fuel for my resentment of authority figures. On top of this, I was hit with a laundry list of charges, including felony DWI, unauthorized license plates, fleeing the scene, no insurance, no driver's license, etc. My teaching job would be finished.

I was actually allowed to bail out on Saturday, posting $12,000 bail—I had to come up with $1200 cash. I spent the next month walking on egg-shells, wondering when it was going to end up in the paper, as I knew that would be the end of me. The anguish I felt walking down to Silver Lake Foods to check the paper on a daily basis will never leave me. The inevitable came about three weeks later, as my charges showed up in the paper. I received a lot of phone calls, and the next day, I was told to resign and leave immediately or be fired. The superintendent of Rochester's Public Schools showed up to give me the news in front of the Burr Oak Staff. I was done. I will never forget Mr. Norlander, the school principal, giving me a ride home that day. Not a word was said. It was eerie. I was done as a teacher and to this day, I have not taught. In the famous words of my father, "You blew it." It was at this time that my life really disintegrated. I was facing felony DWI charges, which had already been plastered all over the paper (people still read papers back then). I was living by myself, and there was no way I was going to be able to afford to keep renting this house with my job as a bookseller (seven-fifty per hour). I also had a blossoming crack cocaine habit and progressive alcoholism. The solution: start to steal from my employer. The DaVinci Code was HUGE back in spring, 2004, and we couldn't keep the book on the shelf. The book was $24.95, and with tax, it was a total of $26.70. Utilizing my math skills, I figured I could ring up four to eight newspapers per night instead of the book and glean $100-$200 from the place. That would give me $104.80, or $209.60, which would buy me crack cocaine and alcohol. It worked out for about three months, and then I was caught, as I became careless, and my till started being off. They brought down an agent that is involved with loss protection, and I was summoned to the office. She stated that there was a camera in a pen and that it showed me taking money out of the register. Now, being a sensible person, cameras in pens are far-fetched. But...take a guy who was up most of the night smoking crack, and cameras in pens are very real. I caved and admitted to the theft. I was arrested after admitted to stealing over $1,000. I probably stole well more than that, but that's the amount they wanted me to admit to. They took me to jail, and my bond was forfeited. I was back in jail again on August 24th.

I sat in intake for about ten days, getting over to the "main popula-tion" on the Sunday of Labor Day weekend. I remember this for multiple reasons, the main one being that I could feel the tension in the room imme-diately upon getting there. The jail was packed, with probably a hundred inmates in a jail that held eighty. People that had single rooms were having to give their space to someone, albeit temporarily, due to overcrowding. This was incredibly stupid, and Olmsted County paid the price. On Labor Day, after brunch at 10:30 am, the inmates revolted. Of course, being a hol-iday, the jail was short staffed, and the inmates started and continued a riot that would become the biggest riot ever in Olmsted County, costing well over one million dollars in damage. Two jailers were forced out of the unit, and the unit was locked. The main switchboard was immediately destroyed as people urinated on it from the upstairs landing. The vending machines were destroyed, toilets were plugged, computers and televisions were smashed to bits, and the chaos ensued for eight or nine hours. I stayed in my room and started writing a letter, stating that this might end up being a big deal. When law enforcement finally broke into the jail in the early evening hours, they were pissed. Many of them were called away from family gatherings, BBQs, etc., to come and round up these adult criminals who were destroying their jail. Upon entering, they shot any inmate walking around outside of their cell with a bean bag that put them down. The toilets had all plugged, and the water level was about one foot in my cell. We were all strip searched and taken to intake cells or empty women's cells. I was taken to intake and sat there for one month, getting out one hour per day to shower and make phone calls. The meals were identical for the entire month—cold and tasteless. One of the jailers came in to see me about two weeks after the riots and told me that he watched the entire tape of my cell and that I only peeked my head out once. I was not going to be given any new charges, which my attorney stated was the smartest thing I had done in years. They asked me if I wanted to see an investigator to "rat" out some of the offenders. I didn't feel right about that, as it was not going to affect me in any way whatsoever. I still had a huge problem with authority and was still blaming everyone but me for my alcoholism, which was a resentment I was certainly not letting go of at that time. I thought treatment would be better than sitting in here, so I put in a kite for an assessment. I vividly remember my CD assessment while I was in solitary confinement, and not because it was this moment of truth where I bared myself to the assessor and had an awakening. It was the way the assessor completed it. His name was "RD," and he probably had done as many assessments at that point as I have over the past twelve years. I was excited to talk to another human, so I went down there with a jump in my gait. I can tell you with clarity that he was cold, callous, and never made eye contact with me over the course of the eighteen-page assessment. It took fifteen minutes, and he was off. He did not give one shit about me as a person, and it felt demeaning. However, I was used to that by now, as shame had become a big part of my life. The good news...I was furloughed to treatment in St. Peter after twenty-six days in solitary, and was on my way to my first inpatient treatment ever.

I took it seriously and tried to get everything I could out of it. I was acting "as if" due to being able to get out of jail and come to Johnson Hall in St. Peter for treatment. I met some cool people and begged my counselor for extra days, as I was getting funded for twenty-one. He called the county for me, and I was given three extra days, which would put me back in jail on a Friday, with sentencing the following Monday. I had to be driven back to the jail after treatment (this is what a furlough means), so Debbie and her parents came to get me on Friday morning. Deb was a total wreck, throwing up in the bathroom of the treatment center and then puking onto the dreamcatcher I made her in treatment. We got back to Rochester, and this was the first time I had been home in about seventy days. I had about two hours before having to report, so we were intimate, and then I took the lonely walk to the jail. Upon arriving, defeated once again, the jailer looked up my information and told me that I did not have to report back to the jail as I initially thought, but "better show up for court Monday, or you will have a warrant put out for your arrest." I was ecstatic, as I had about seventy days sober, felt good, and thought I would have a wonderful weekend with Deb SOBER!!! However, she had other plans, and I returned home to bikes in the yard, people in the house partying, and alcohol and drugs everywhere. My old crack dealer was lounging around in there, along with several other guys I did not know. I immediately grabbed my dog and walked up to a gas station, and called my friend Will, who came and picked me up. I spent the weekend at his home sober. I showed up for court on Monday and was sentenced for both the felony DWI and the felony theft. I received 180 days in jail for the DWI, 145 days in jail for the theft but was given the sentences concurrent (meaning I only had to do the 180 in jail) and was given the work release option. They "hung" thirty-six months in prison over my head in case I managed to mess this up. I didn't have high hopes for myself, even with a little sobriety. I also got two big FELONIES on my record, which cost me a lot in my recovery (much more on that later). I was to report the Monday after Thanksgiving, so I had three weeks before another return trip to jail. I spent the next three weeks sober and reported to jail on November 29th, 2004, with over ninety days of sobriety. With credit for time already served and STS days worked, I was released on February 11th, 2005. I worked twenty-one days of "sentence to serve" county work, where I would work eight hours on a crew for a day off the back end of my sentence. I also was able to find employment at Andy's liquor during the three weeks between treatment and jail, so I had a job to go to five days per week. This was good and bad. The good was that I felt like I was part of the human race during the time I spent in jail, but the bad news was that I was around alcohol every day (and I was not supposed to be working a job that served or sold alcohol). I had to call from next door at an insurance company (told them I cleaned the place) and hoped they wouldn't show up one day to "check on me." Being around alcohol every day did not affect me while I was incarcerated (so I thought), but it affected me down the road. I managed to stay sober for a few months once I was released, and I did this by going to AA meetings and working with a sponsor. I had gone to AA sporadically over the past four or five years, but only to get a card signed for probation. I was working a program and had been sober since my incarceration in August, so I had some time under my belt. Deb was trying too, but she never really stopped drinking. I was around alcohol daily with my job, and people I knew from my sordid past started coming in to buy liquor, including someone that sold crack cocaine. Having it in your home environment, working around it forty hours per week, and then having people you know come in and buy liquor and ask you to buy drugs became too much to bear. I set up my relapse methodically, with the July 4th weekend in mind. July 4th fell on a Sunday, and that meant Monday was a vacation day for me. I bought an eight ball of crack on July 1st from someone who shorted me (it was one gram, but I didn't care) and eight bottles of Budweiser aluminum pints. These sat in the garage along with the crack for two days, and there were many times when I had the chance to talk to someone and have them come over and help me dispose of them. After all, I had made a lot of friends in AA. However, the choice was made in my head about two weeks prior to the holiday, and there was ultimately no turning back. I can't imagine how much dopamine was released every time I thought about what was sitting in the garage those two days prior to my relapse. This was not an impulsive relapse but was methodically planned for weeks. My sobriety totaled ten and a half months, my relapse lasted twenty-two months, and I scraped the bottom of the proverbial barrel with this one.

That first relapse opened up all of the pleasure receptors in my brain, and I got bad fast. I started drinking at work, drinking daily, and smoking as much crack as I could. I started to fall behind on my bills, which had become a trend of mine in the past due to the cost of crack and my obsession with it. I began spending time at Olympic Village apartments with a "friend" I met in jail that sold crack. He was on EHM for alcohol but smoked and sold crack. My relationship with crack cocaine became an obsession of mine, and I was chasing that euphoria of the first "bell ringer" as I unloaded my money to the dealers at a fever pitch. This was my version of "chasing the dragon," as I found myself looking for the "feeling" I got with that first hit. The problem is, you never get it again, and that is the obsession and compulsion to do hard drugs. Crack gave me euphoria like nothing else, including methamphetamine. I would smoke it and run around Rochester naked in the middle of the night, acting without a care in the world. This was my new "drug of choice," and it was also my kryptonite. It was nothing for me to smoke three to five grams in an evening, which would force me to steal from my employer once again. I was getting careless at work and paranoid that people were going to find me out and I was going to go back to jail or prison. The day finally came when I was fired at the liquor store; they said they found out I had two felonies. I don't believe this; I think they realized someone was stealing from the place, and saw that I had a felony for stealing from an employer. I was done there in October of 2005, about three months after relapsing.

The Nursery Experience

I had had several conversations with the owner of a landscape company over the course of my time at the liquor store, as he was a Friday customer about once per month. He was a really good guy and talked about his business with passion. I knew he sold Christmas trees at Crossroads shopping center and so I went down and asked him for a job. He hired me and told me that if I did a good job selling Christmas trees, there might be a winter job for me that would get me to spring, where his business really takes off. I accepted and started around the nursery, cleaning and waiting to go and get the trees from several tree farms. I was selling Christmas trees daily from mid-November to Christmas Eve. He appreciated my work, and it moved into 2006, when I was putting wires on pots for hanging plants. I then moved into selling bare root trees for him and created some new accounts. He started mentoring me and talking to me more and more about the nursery business. I had officially rebounded from another lost job and got smug over time. I found out where they kept the cash from the sales at the nursery, and again, this became my downfall. He was so good to me, and I took advantage of his trust. They gave me a car to drive every night, even though I did not have a driver's license. I worked around the nursery once spring hit, selling trees, working in the yard, selling mulch, whatever I could do. Saturdays were crazy days for sales once flowers bloomed, and I worked weekends. My crack cocaine habit was also in full bloom, as well as ongoing drinking. I found a credit card in the vehicle they were letting me drive, and I started using that to buy money for phone cards, which I gave to the dealers for crack. I started doing this in the summer, and it actually lasted until September 2006. I went to use the card, and it had been canceled. I was told I could not drive a vehicle the next day. I was then called two days later and told I was done, but I could come and get my last check, which I did. The owner looked at me with some pity, and I walked away, shameful, and jobless once again. Two weeks later, I received a document in the mail stating that I was being investigated for theft, but this eventually dissolved, and I heard through one of his employees that it was due to the cost of taking someone to court. Oh, well, I continued to put my college degree to good use and started working at Little Caesars Pizza and was hired almost immediately.

"I Will Deny My Role…as a Human"

I was plunging to new depths with my drug use and "settling" on jobs that were beneath the standard of someone who had been a teacher and coach. However, I didn't care. I was able to utilize my math skills to figure out how to steal one-hundred dollars per night from there. A "hot-n-ready" pizza was $5.35 with tax, and so four of them added up to $21.40. If I were to not ring up twenty pizzas per night, it would total $107. This was enough to get me a gram of crack. So…if someone came in and paid for two pizzas, I would see that they were paying cash and then ring up one. If they bought four, I would ring up two. This worked great on Friday and Saturday nights, as there were football games, which meant football parties. Well, as with anything illegal, this was not going to last. Once I had the $100, I would call my dealer, and he would pull up, and I would run him out a cheese pizza with $100 inside the box. He would give me the crack, and the deal would be done. The inevitable was bound to happen, and it certainly did. I came into work one day, and there were signs up everywhere that stated, "We have a thief in the house." Pizza boxes were counted, and there was a huge shortage. No one was allowed on the tills anymore except managers. However, I was able to talk the weeknight manager Pete into allowing me limited access to the till. I continued to steal small amounts until one day I came in, and the manager told me that I was being let go, and he gave me no further explanation. There would be no charges here, but again, I was without a job. I had made it there three months, and I was reaching the end of the line. I mean, when you get fired from Little Caesar's Pizza, you know you are starting to scrape the bottom of the barrel. I was going to end up in prison or dead. I started dumpster diving after Little Caesar's closed because I had no food in the fridge. I subsisted on "cold and ready's" for a month or so. To make things even worse, I couldn't pay the rent anymore, and my landlord, who had called me the best renter he ever had in 2003, now called me "the biggest piece of shit he had ever met." He stated that he didn't care about the back rent he just wanted me out. I made plans to move on February 14th, 2007, and moved my stuff to the basement of a house I found to rent about five blocks away. I had been looking for employment following the loss of my job and found part-time work at a pet store and daily work at Reichel Foods through Labor Ready. These two jobs were enough to get me some money to pay for my security deposit and first month's rent.

I remember actually thinking that this was going to work out, which showed how far I had regressed. My job at Reichel Foods was through Labor Ready, where you showed up at 5:30 am to get temporary work. I got in at Reichel Foods on a 6:00 am-2:00 pm gig, where I proceeded to snap lids on meat and cheese trays for eight hours per day. I worked between two Asian gentlemen that didn't speak a lick of English. There were no windows. It was a horrible job, and it paid me forty-seven dollars per day. This gave me a crack rock each day, which I would smoke up in about five minutes. Hell of a trade-off!! This also meant that I would be looking to con and hustle for more, which meant I would not show up for work the next morning. This meant I had to go back to Labor Ready and get back on the list for Reichel. It was an absolutely miserable experience. The job at "Fish-n-Pets" did not last long either, as one day I came into work and saw my hours were reduced. There were no reasons given. Then I was off the schedule and terminated. I was boxed into a corner and really started to lose hope for myself. I was really progressing in crack use, which resulted in some scary changes inside of me. I pawned a lot of my sports memorabilia, but for some reason, I did not pawn my stereo equipment, which should show you how much music means to me. The two girls that lived upstairs were "afraid of me," according to the landlord. My crack addiction had made me into less than a human, and it had possessed me in the worst way possible. I saw no way out of this mess until the fateful morning when I had an awakening and a moment of clarity.

The Life Had Taken Enough from Me – Time for a Change

The evening before the "fateful morning" in question was like many of my crack cocaine-fueled evenings —I stayed up most of the night smoking crack, cleaning the pipe, smoking crack resin, riding my bike around town, etc. I remember lying down, and my heart was beating so fast that I became mesmerized by it. I asked God to take me, to just make my heart burst. I eventually must have fallen asleep for a couple of hours because after I woke up late for work again, I was walking amongst the carnage of the night before and found fifty cents. I remember looking at it and thinking how odd it was that I would have this laying around, as I normally spent everything I had on crack (even the change). I took this down to a pay phone and called Olmsted County Social Services and set up an assessment for some time in mid-May. I believe there was a two-week wait time to get into inpatient treatment, and in that period of time, I drank several times and smoked crack exactly one time, as I was owed some money from Reichel Foods/Labor Ready. Other than that, I just kind of waited for this opportunity to go and get help. I had a sense of calm around me during that time, and I moved all of my possessions into my parent's house the day I left. My mother and father actually drove me to treatment that day and gave me a card to read for when I was there. They were being supportive, which I didn't feel I deserved. I entered Fountain Center's inpatient treatment program on May 25th, 2007, and took a clean urine screen. My sobriety journey (unbeknownst to me) had begun.

The Carnage Summarized –
The Years of Incarceration

This is probably the perfect spot to talk about my years spent incarcerated, as my criminal record has followed me around and created a lot of stress and angst over the years. To summarize...I picked up five DWIs from 1987-2004 (1987, 1994, 1999, 2000, 2004), the last one being a felony. Due to my alcoholism and drug addiction, I spent roughly 1,000 days incarcerated from 1999-2005. This six-year time period was spent in and out of jail, collecting DWIs like I used to collect baseball cards, driving without a license, driving without insurance, and once I started my crack cocaine habit, theft. Jail was becoming my norm, and I started to get used to that routine. I have been in three different county jails, including Winona, Olmsted, and Carver County. I found it started getting easy to go to jail, and that scared me a little. I was becoming a "frequent flyer," as some of the jailers called me. One particular judge would say to me, "What are we going to do with you today, Mr. Volz?" I would reply, "I can do thirty days in jail standing on my head." Her retort back, "Well then, we are going to give you sixty days to get back on your feet again." Very amusing. Other charges I incurred over this time included a disorderly conduct in Cannon Falls when I hurled a hubcap through one of the town businesses after staggering out of the Yellow Bird bar drunk. I also had two theft convictions, one being a felony. I received three driving after cancellations, as I was "inimical to public safety." This means that I was deemed to pose too great a risk to others to allow me to continue driving. I bring all of this to the reader's attention because this criminal record was what I was faced with after I got sober and made the decision to go back to school to advance and enhance my career. I didn't know if I was going to have a career, as I had dug myself a deep hole and on some days, I did not think there was going to be a future. I always knew that my criminal record was going to be an albatross for me and a permanent target on my back. It certainly has not helped me after getting sober, and to be honest, it has been the biggest stressor I have had to endure. I totally understand why people relapse when they are not allowed to move forward in their lives, and the stigma of who they used to be remains a constant battle. To this day, there are people in the professional field who see me and do not see the person that has overcome but the person I used to be. This no longer haunts me like it used to, but to be honest, it has taken its toll. I have had to work a strong program of recovery in order to work as a counselor in recovery, and as you read on, you will see why. This criminal past I carry around has been my biggest burden, bar none, as I have had to relive it over and over again. It is a stigmatizing brand that sizzles on your forehead. It has gotten easier, but it is still there. It has certainly closed many doors permanently, and maybe after reading the last fifty pages, you think it is something I deserve. However, if you continue reading, I think you will see that I have tried hard every day to make up for "the years of decay."

There were some positives coming out of the years of incarceration, although it takes a lot to see that, even today. The first positive was that every trip to jail was one step closer to getting sober. Without consequences, most people will not seek help, let alone get sober. I had a lot of legal consequences, and they all added up in the end. They took their toll on me from an emotional perspective, and the body kept the score. The other positive I can see out of the years of incarceration has to do with my sobriety. I was able to garner some sober time in jail (well, when I wasn't in work release), and it stopped me from continuing my use. Most importantly, the sober time felt good. This might have saved me as my risky behaviors progressed with my alcohol and drug use. Those forced periods of sobriety might have saved my life. Thanks, Linda!!

PART II

The Road to Redemption

The Friday afternoon of Memorial Day weekend was the beginning of my second inpatient treatment and seventh overall attempt (I had attempted five different outpatient programs but do not remember completing any of them). I was to go to FC in Albert Lea, and I arrived around 4:00 pm. I got there in time for dinner, met some of my peers, and got settled in. I did not meet my counselor until after I was there for five days. I spent the first four days there playing cards and attending one meeting. My assignments were all shared on one day in group, and they were all based on my non-existing relationship with my daughter (that has changed). I did not have any say in the treatment plan at all. My friend wrote a letter to FC and told them I was basically a piece of garbage, which didn't help much. That was read in front of the group, which was shaming and incredibly hurtful. I was there for twenty-one days total, which went by incredibly fast. But…the food was good, and the Ulstad building in Albert Lea was a great place for AA. Having stated all this about my experience at FC, I also must say I am blessed and grateful to have had the opportunity to go there. It was exactly what I needed, even though it was only three weeks. I was able to get back into reality a little bit, ate well, exercised well, prayed in the chapel every day, and went to education groups, AA groups, and treatment groups. It was what I made it, and it was the start I needed. It was also the second time I was given a "free ride" by the state of Minnesota. I was given twenty-four days in treatment in 2004 and twenty-one days in treatment this time, and I am eternally grateful for both of those opportunities.

I did not get a medallion when I graduated but instead, was given a camel pin. My counselor stated that if I went to aftercare for three months at FC in Rochester, he would give me a medallion. I did that more because I did not think he gave me much of a chance to stay sober, and I wanted to prove him wrong (proving people wrong has been a constant source of motivation for me throughout my sobriety journey). I left FC a little scared exactly three weeks after getting dropped off there and was given a ride back to Rochester by one of their staff. The driver dropped me off at an AA meeting in Rochester on Friday at 1:00 pm. I walked in late with my suitcases and sat down next to Deb, who stated she was going to be there. She reeked of booze. I opened my mouth and started to share about just getting out of inpatient treatment and someone piped up, "We are happy for you, but until you get a sponsor and work the steps, we would appreciate it if you kept your mouth shut." WOW—I was not expecting that. My poor ego was bruised right off the bat. I fought the urge to leave the meeting right then and there, but something kept me in that seat. I went to a meeting the next morning at another club and got another white chip (and a sponsor) and went back for more "abuse" at the Pioneer Club the following Monday. I was back in the community and suiting up and showing up! I started going to meetings daily and found several that worked for me. That 1:00 pm meeting was a crazy meeting, with some serious chronic alcoholics in there. However, that is what I needed. It was hardcore. After working the twelve steps with my temporary sponsor, I found a permanent sponsor, and we met at noon on Mondays before the meeting. I found employment at Taco John's and a pizza place and started to save money. Taco John's came about in a weird way, as I must have applied there before going to inpatient treatment because they called my parent's house three days after getting out of treatment and wanted an interview. I took the interview and accepted the job for eight dollars per hour. This was one of my "jobs of humility" that I took that really turned out to be a great decision.

Living at my parent's house, riding a bicycle, and working at Taco John's at the age of thirty-nine should probably seem humiliating, and maybe sometimes I felt that way, especially because I was living with my parents, riding a bicycle, and working at Wendy's when I was seventeen! However, most of the time, I felt a large dose of gratitude due to my sobriety, my parents allowing me to stay there, and the people I began to meet in the recovery community. I had been given a chance, and using any drugs or alcohol now was a choice, not the necessity I thought it was when in the middle of my long run. I embraced feeling better, and I attacked the one-mile-long hill with vigor when returning home from work. I talked to my folks daily, kept my nose to the grindstone, and tried not to think too much about the future. I forged a relationship with my parents for the first time ever, I think. I kept things simple and adopted a minimalist attitude. This relationship with my parents allowed me to let go of a lot of the pent-up resentment I held toward my mother. I worked at Taco John's forty hours per week, worked at a pizza joint twelve hours per week, attended one meeting daily, lived at my parent's house, and rode my bicycle. That's what I did. That was my first six months of sobriety. I found a sponsor, and started working the steps. I did not have a phone, so I had minimal temptations. I did not tell anyone where I lived and just focused hard on building sober days. Meanwhile, three guys I got close to in treatment all relapsed, and they tried to drag me into it. My parents saved my ass that night, and they had no clue what living there did for me over the first ninety days after treatment. I found a house for rent after about ninety days at my parents and moved in on October 1st. This place was owned by the family of a guy I was in treatment with, and it was a nice place. The only problem was they were not paying the mortgage, and it went into foreclosure. I was served the papers about six months after moving in. However, there was a house right next to this one that appeared to be empty, and an old man would come over and mow the grass every now and then. I went over and talked to him and found out that he lived with his "girlfriend," and this house was indeed empty. I asked him if he would let me move in there, and he finally acquiesced for $500 per month. I lived there for four years. They say that good things happen when you are doing the right things, and this I have found to be true. I had never really wanted sobriety before, and this time felt different. In the past, there was always an external factor playing in my "forced" sobriety, such as a probation officer, a new crime, etc. This is "artificial motivation," and that didn't work for me. I spent most of my previous sober time incarcerated, other than the time in 2004-2005 when I made it over four months after my jail stint. This time, I felt like I had a hand in my decision to get well, as I went into treatment on my own. That made a big difference. Also, I was thirty-nine years old and felt like if I didn't get it soon, I would miss out on fulfilling my potential (whatever that was). I was also tired of this way of life; crack cocaine and alcohol had led me to a life of isolation and loneliness, the likes of which I would never wish on anyone. I didn't want anyone to see me this way, so I lived in the shadows, avoiding anyone who may have known me. But. . . not at Taco John's. There I was in the midst of many humans and worked the infamous Taco Tuesday, where soft shell tacos were one dollar. It was here where I had my first God moment, so to speak. It was a little test, and although I certainly did not know it at the time, it was a stepping stone to becoming a more honest person and learning the value of integrity.

It was a typical Tuesday at Taco John's, and the line stretched almost out the door. We had extra people working every Tuesday afternoon to help with the crazy lunch rush we were hit with from about 11:30 am to 1:30 pm. It was around noon, and I was working the Steak Escape Grill side, as this Taco John's location also included a second restaurant. I looked out at the swarm of humans and saw two former teaching colleagues standing in line. They had not seen me yet, but I immediately got anxious and felt a deep sense of shame. I thought of my options: Run to the back and hide for fifteen minutes, leave and never come back, ignore them, and hope they don't see me, or face them and talk to them. I bring this up because this is one of those big moments that can propel you forward in your recovery journey or bring you back to the insanity of addiction. I don't know what overcame me, but I told myself I was done running away and I walked up to them both and extended my hand. They both shook it and asked how I was doing. I told them, "I am right where I need to be right now." I then went back and assumed my station. The feeling of calm that embraced me was stunning. It was my higher power telling me I just did the right thing and that everything was going to be all right. It was a powerful moment for me and one that I will never forget. It was also around this time that I no longer cared what other people thought of me. It was liberating, and it allowed me to speak up for myself, and unbeknownst to me, something I did for my clients later on in my journey.

My toiling at Taco John's and Uncle G's pizza did not last long, as Uncle G's closed and I started to look for better employment in late 2007. I was hired at a place called Paradise Pete's and was the pizza side manager. I was given a salary akin to about twelve dollars an hour, but this was a decent raise for me, and I accepted. The pizza side was busy, as the place had a reputation for having amazing pizza going back to when it was called Pizza Man. The owners were alcoholics and loved the Jimmy Buffet experience of drunken "hippydom," so they turned their restaurant into a tropical paradise, with surfboards on the wall, palm trees, rock gardens with waterfalls, and a menu that catered to that theme. It was all disguised so they could drink all day. I worked Tuesday through Saturday from 2:00 pm to 12:00 pm and had Sundays and Mondays off. This allowed me to get to my meetings, meet with my sponsor, and stay busy on the weekends. The Winter of 2007-2008 was overwhelmingly busy, especially on the weekends. Pizzas were going out of the restaurant at a fever pitch, and the fast-paced atmosphere was good for me. That structure and routine was much needed for me, as I was an alcoholic and a stimulant addict, and I needed to be busy—very busy.

I got my six-month sobriety coin in November and was carving out a recovery routine. This was mainly due to Alcoholics Anonymous, as I had never had that length of sobriety outside of jail. I found a sponsor at my first AA meeting at Tradition III, and worked the steps in about two months. This was the first time I worked them with no reservation, and my fourth and fifth steps were done with fearlessness. After we finished step nine, my sponsor told me we were done (he committed to being my temporary sponsor), and he recommended I find another one at Pioneer Club, which turned out to be my home group and club until 2020 when I switched things up and found a new home group. I did what he asked, found a pastor at the 1:00 pm meeting, and we met weekly and once again went through the *Big Book*. I was at the point in my life where I was willing to take suggestions, which is why this worked for me. Alcohol and crack cocaine had stopped working years before I quit, and I just wanted a different life. I stopped thinking so much about the future and just embraced the day, living in the moment and building a new foundation. That is what the first three years were all about. I had no idea what God had in store for me at that time—I just became a recovery "grinder," trudging through day after day. This life was so much better than my old life, which was filled with anxiety, fear, bitterness, isolation, and the "four horsemen" they talk about in the *Big Book*—Terror, Bewilderment, Frustration, and Despair. Looking back today, I guess I was reveling in the simplicity of my life at the age of thirty-nine. As long as I stayed sober, a new life would be laid out for me. I thought I knew what it was going to be, but "I plan, God laughs" It turned out a lot different than I thought it would be.

The Winter Bike Riding Experiment

Imoved into a house close to my home AA club, but I had to bike everywhere else. That meant biking during the Minnesota winters, which are brutal and show no remorse. I was still three years away from getting my driver's license back, and riding my bike became one more lesson in humility for me (and, I have to admit, some humiliation). I was putting on twenty-twenty-five miles per day, and this was very beneficial to my overall physical health. However, the winter is a tough row to hoe, and I had to put on layer after layer and make sure to avoid icy patches. It might seem like a small feat, but pushing forty years old and riding a cheap mountain bike in the winter will give you some gratitude for being able to drive. I don't take any of that for granted today because I spent ages thirty-nine to forty-one on my bike, and that helped me gain integrity and personal growth. Riding that old bike taught me another big lesson as well, and that was to not take the easy way out. I know a lot of people who get sober but are still "living dirty." They continue to take "small permissions" with their sobriety, such as driving without a driver's license. I did not want to play that game; I wanted to do things the right way. Most of the time, the right way is the hard way, and that is important to point out. I had used alcohol and drugs for most of the past twenty-two years, and the only way I was going to make the changes was to do things by the book. I could not cheat my sobriety—I would not have stayed the course if I had taken shortcuts.

Winter turned to spring, and Paradise Pete's stayed busy until the summer and then slowed down. Weekends were still relatively busy for pizza delivery, but the restaurant sales were way down, and weeknights were very slow. The owners began to start growling a little bit as their business went from rolling in the money to being slow, and they didn't really know how to handle this. I was working in a place where I was counting money in the bar at 1:00 am, and there was liquor everywhere. The owners reeked of it by the end of the night, and they would stop to talk on their way out the door, triggering me with liquor on their breath. There were times when I was counting money and ringing out the till, and I would have to get on my knees and pray, as there were Summer Shandy's on ice ten feet away from me (I still have never tried that one). There were some hard nights, and after a while, I just needed a change. I hung on there longer than I should have and finally left in the fall of 2008. In the interim, some rewards of my sobriety over the summer included getting off probation and making it to one year of sobriety.

One Year Sober

I vividly remember a video they would play in one of my outpatient treatment episodes about a guy going to get his one-year cake, and he was reliving memories about the events leading up to this day. This included falls down stairs, DWIs, fogginess, family quarrels, etc. I sat there and watched it thinking, *There is no way I am ever going to get to one year sober. It will never happen.* I think I watched the video three or four times, or each time I was admitted to their facility. Well, eight years after watching that silly videotape, my day had arrived. It was May 25th, 2008, and I had hit one year of sobriety. I bought myself a nice forty-inch big screen TV as a gift to myself, and still have that today. I remember getting my one-year coin, but I cannot remember what I said. I focused hard on continuing my sobriety, as I was feeling good, and I was driven. Someone once said, "Pray for a slow recovery." I know what that means today, and that was monumental in my early recovery. I had a high ceiling and had a long way to go, and that drove me. I had attended an AA meeting almost every day for the first eighteen months, and found a nice home group meeting, where I started meeting good people. I attended sober functions, got heavily involved in the fellowship, worked the twelve steps, and stayed busy. I received a letter in the mail sometime in April or May, stating I had completed my probation in Olmsted County. I had actually forgotten I was still on probation and didn't have any responsibilities to it. However, the letter was well received and needed once I began the process of trying to resurrect my career. I lived recovery, and the jobs I held were not ones that I would have to take home with me —they were relatively stress-free. In a nutshell, I was moving away from my past and building a foundation for my future. The first year of sobriety was extremely hard, but due to my willingness to accept some jobs of humility, it was somewhat stress-free. I don't know if I could have done it any other way. I had to change twenty-two years of habits, routines, and ingrained alcoholic thinking. This was no small feat, but I think all my years playing sports laid a good foundation for the discipline I needed that first year. I needed a lot of grit, discipline, and mental toughness, which still drive me today.

Savers and RSD #535 - Curveballs

I started thinking about getting back into substitute teaching in the fall of 2008, and these thoughts led me to Saver's, where I applied for a part-time night job. My days of bartending to supplement my teaching were over, so I needed to find something close to where I lived. I got hired there in September of 2008 as a part-time evening worker and made my move to get back into the school district. Paradise Pete's received my two-week notice in early November, and I went to the substitute teacher orientation in the middle of that month. I was making some changes that would benefit my life and recovery, or so I thought. When I got in front of a hundred people at the end of November and received my eighteen-month sobriety coin, I told them all these things that I was going to do, including teaching, coaching, and moving forward in my life. Little did I know that there was another plan in store for me and hard life lessons to learn.

I went to the orientation for substitute teachers and received my badge/name tag. I was given a code to enter when calling the "sub finder" for jobs and was told to wait one day for it to become active. I had experience with substitute teaching in Rochester, and this was going to be a good thing for me, I thought. Two days later, it was still inactive. I called the Edison Building/Human Resources, and they told me that the Director of Human Resources needed to have a conversation with me, and we made an appointment for a Friday after Thanksgiving weekend. I got in there, and as soon as I sat down in her office, I got this sick feeling in my stomach—one that I would have many more times as I attempted to navigate back into some semblance of a professional career. My criminal record had reared its ugly head (this would become something that followed me around for the past fifteen years like a plague), and the HR person told me, "We cannot have you teaching in the school district because you have two felonies. What if a parent of one of the students you were teaching found out a multiple felon was standing in front of their child? We cannot have you teach in ISD #535. You can try at some of the other districts." I struggled with my acceptance of this, and my first thoughts of using in months glimmered to the surface. My mother had given me a ride to the meeting, and she took me home. She did not want to leave me, as she had a legitimate fear I was going to throw away eighteen months of sobriety. Truth be told, I did not know what I was going to do, but after she left, I started legging it down to Crossroads Shopping Center to either go beg for full-time hours at Savers or hit Andy's Liquor Store. I was already looking for ways to justify a relapse, as I had not played the tape forward or played out all the scenarios. At eighteen months, I was still pretty sick and thought that since I had gotten sober, all of my past would just dissipate. It was still right there, and it was rearing its ugly head for the first time since I had gotten sober. I was running on anger and resentment at this point, and alcohol was a real option for me at this time. This was another one of those moments that would be instrumental and crucial in my recovery. It might be the most important one of all because I think it was one of the last times I really craved a drink or drug.

I started hoofing it and hit the Crossroads parking lot. I remember there was a nursery that set up shop in the corner of the lot every year to sell Christmas trees, and I approached the corner of the lot, thirst building, anger boiling, resentment engulfing me. A car rolled by, and the driver rolled down the window. It was "Karen" from the Monday 4:30 Promises Meeting at Methodist Hospital. "How are you doing?" she asked. "Fine," I replied, and happy holidays and all that shit. She drove off, and I continued my walk through the lot. A second vehicle drove up and rolled down the window. It was someone from my Sunday morning AA meeting — "Hey, Tim. How goes it?" "Fine," I state, and off he goes. I hit the sidewalk that will take me to the liquor store, and a guy comes walking out of one of the stores. He often chaired the 1:00 pm meeting at the Pioneer, and we knew each other. "Hey, Tim!!!" he bellowed. "How are you doing?" Well, the third time was the charm for me because I told him I was not well and that I was very angry, resentful, bitter, frustrated, etc. He offered me a ride around, and I told him what had happened. He listened to me and took it all in. He told me to go to that night's AA meeting at 7:00 pm and talk about it, process it, and move forward. I did exactly that. This was my first spiritual experience, as God meticulously placed three people in my path on that cold, snowy day because he knows I am a slow learner. It just couldn't be one or two—it had to be three. The connections I had made in the first eighteen months of sobriety had saved my butt, and a couple of weeks later, I called Winona State and started in their new addictions counseling program. My first class started in the summer of 2009. Oh, and by the way, I was hired full-time at Saver's and found employment next door to Saver's at the Dollar Tree. Two more "jobs of humility" that helped to shape who I was becoming.

Learning the Gift of Minimalism
With Two Jobs of Humility

I began working in the back room at Saver's, sorting roughly eight thousand pounds of cloth each day and met some wild characters in my time back there. This was a felon-friendly place, so there were many active drug addicts working and using there. It was a meth party every day back there for some people, who were wide-eyed and paranoid of their own shadow. It was a riot. I met my friend Randy there, who was on parole, and one of the most institutionalized people I have ever met. He spent sixteen years in prison for a crime committed in a blackout when he was in his teens. He did not like people, but he did like heavy music, and that was what bonded us. We are friends to this day and have attended about twenty concerts together. Our first concert together was Goatwhore, The Berserker, and Warbringer in 2009, and the last one we attended was in February of 2020, where we took in the Polish death metal band Vader.

When May rolled around, I hit the two-year mark of sobriety, and I continued my routine of attending meetings. I started hitting two or three per week, after hitting one per day for the first eighteen months. My schedule had changed as well, as I began taking graduate classes through Winona State's new Addictions Counseling Program. My schedule looked like this: Monday through Friday at Savers from 8:00 am to 5:00 pm, Dollar Tree Mondays 5:00 pm to 9:00 pm, Thursdays 5:00 pm to 9:00 pm, and Saturdays 7:00 am to 4:00 pm, and Tuesday and Wednesday at WSU from 6:00 pm to 9:00 pm. Sundays were my study days. This busy schedule was something that became almost an afterthought over the next twelve years, as my time became crunched around all my responsibilities, as well as the character defect of thinking I had to make up for all the lost time during my active years of addiction. But I digress—I got busy and started to find my purpose and passion by going back to school. This gave me some hope as well that my life was moving in the right direction.

The Dollar Tree was a job that allowed me to stock shelves for four to eight hours three times per week, and it was an easy job that I have a lot of gratitude for, even today. My willingness to take these jobs of humility back in early recovery has helped me so much later on in my continued personal growth. I know many people who would scoff at taking a shelf stocking job at the age of forty; I saw this with some clients who didn't want to "lower their standards." However, these were the same people who would relapse on meth for four straight days until they went into psychosis. The Dollar Tree provided no stress, and between this job and Saver's, my employment allowed me to focus on my recovery. When school started in May of 2009 I was two years clean, and ready for a challenge. This came at a perfect time for me; remember the "slow recovery" mantra? Yeah, that was me. Slow like a tortoise.

The Return of the College Student at Forty-One

I began school in 2009 much like an adolescent, riding my bicycle to class. I had no computer, so I needed to carve out time to get to the college and utilize their computer room. I had limited knowledge of computers, other than doing some IEPs when teaching kids with behavior disorders. However, I was a quick learner and became proficient in no time. This gave me a renewed identity, and I began to connect with some of my fellow classmates. I was two years sober, and the shame of riding my bike to class was long gone. I had accepted the road carved out by years of addiction and was very grateful to be given another chance. I put on a lot of miles driving out to the campus for classes and getting on their computers, but I got into a routine. I'd show up at class fresh from Saver's, in my Iron Maiden shirt, and people would be in there with suits and dress clothes after just pushing in their chairs at their office jobs. It was surreal, coming into campus on my bike and showing up for class sweaty but right on time. I belonged there and was paying for these classes out of my own pocket. I have no idea how, but I was able to pay for all of my graduate classes out of pocket until I got to the last two, and received a grant for those six credits. I began to focus hard on balance because I worked forty hours at Saver's, thirteen to sixteen at Dollar Tree, and was taking two classes over the summer, which put me at about eighty hours total for the week. I did not forget about my recovery, but I did start to reduce the number of meetings I was attending each week. I was in the "maintenance" stage of change. Going to school was a sufficient substitute for a meeting every day, as I was enjoying some personal growth and some elevated self-esteem. I was starting the process of making my way back to a second career. . .it was arduous.

I had one more job stop before officially getting into the field of addictions work, and that was at HyVee. This happened around October of 2009, and I made the move from Saver's to HyVee. I was getting nine dollars per hour, which I thought was amazing ($8.41 was my current salary at Saver's). I was ready for a change and made the switch over after about eighteen months at Saver's. I was taking one class in the winter, so I settled into my job in the meat department. Classes continued to go well, and for the first time since I had gotten sober, life appeared to be somewhat normal. I was staying busy, moving up the "proverbial ladder," staying sober, attending meetings, going to school, helping others, and spending time with sober people. I was doing ok and was still working my routine. This continued through into 2010 when I saw an opportunity to work at a sober house for chronic alcoholics and addicts, and I applied at the Cronin Home. I ended up getting the job, and this marked the beginning of my career working in the field of addictions. It was a game changer for me and gave me a daily look at the life of the chronically addicted population. It was like looking in the mirror at what used to be.

825 West Silver Lake Drive

I began working there as a night manager, and worked the 2:00 pm to 10:00 pm shift from Monday through Friday. It paid eleven dollars an hour and was a fast-paced shift, including prepping and serving forty-four residents a homemade dinner and then cleaning the kitchen and dining room after. It was a great job, and I loved it. I was trained to distribute medications to the residents, and I started to absorb everything I could about these medications, including side effects, actions, and when they should be taken. It was my introduction to methadone, anti-depressants, benzos, opioids, mood stabilizers, and ADHD stimulants. I was given a copy of the *2008 Nurse's Medication Handbook* and studied it. I started to learn about harm reduction, which is basically reducing alcohol and drug use, with the goal of increased overall wellness. These residents were "chronic," which meant twenty or more treatments, multiple co-morbid diagnoses, no significant lifetime lengths of sobriety, and a lot of legal stuff and homelessness. I was empathetic and treated them with respect, and soon many were trusting me and spending time in the office talking to me about their stories, and I started asking them about their goals. I was getting the opportunity to work daily with addicts, and I used this platform to start gaining counseling "micro-skills" such as active listening, showing empathy, non-verbal cues, and haptics. I was in the midst of daily crises, and this gave me the chance to work on calming techniques with residents. The Cronin Home taught me a lot about what was to come in the counseling profession. It was a great fit, and my work ethic had grown strong over the years, so I was impressing the brass. I was taking spring classes now and was going to be able to finish the six core classes in the summer of 2010. The one barrier (besides relapse) that could potentially trip me up was the big elephant in the room—my past criminal record. This was something that could not be avoided. I anxiously awaited the day when my background check would come back, and I would be told to walk away from working with vulnerable adults. It was stressful, anxiety-provoking, and traumatic; I held my breath going to the mailbox every day, just as I used to do after getting a DUI. It took months to get back, and in the interim, you worry, and you stress, and it can be the death of someone. The Department of Human Services (DHS) has taken longer than one year to get back to me with their decision on whether or not they will let me work with vulnerable adults, and if they say no, the results can be disastrous for people in recovery. There is a longer section later in this book devoted to that process, and the effects of leaving people in the lurch for that long.

Driving Again and Interning at Fountain Center

I remember going to my interview at Fountain Centers for my internship on my three-year sobriety anniversary on May 25th, 2010. I still hadn't gotten my driver's license back, so I had to get a ride. I was accepted and scheduled to start around mid-August. This gave me the summer to finish my classes, get my driver's license, and get into my new routine at Cronin. I was getting ready to start a "schedule from hell," and it would be the first of many years of being out of balance. I had a strong will and drive to succeed, and grit and mental toughness were traits that I had been compiling during those three years of recovery. As I look back now, the first three years were probably the best three years of my recovery, due to the lack of work-related stress, the effort and time I could put into community recovery, regaining my physical health, and the thrill of the "comeback." I got my driver's license back ten days before I was to start interning. I had gone without a valid license for over ten years, so this was another huge step and advancement for my recovery.

My first day at my internship gave me a glimpse into the field of addictions counseling. I was naïve and thought the atmosphere would be similar to when I was teaching, where people would smile at you, take you under their wing, and treat you with some respect. You know, the apple on the teacher's desk vibe. That was certainly not the case. I got there for my first day and was greeted by the receptionist, who had me complete some paperwork. Once that was completed, I remember going down to the male unit, where I used to be a client. I sat there and reacquainted myself with the place. There was no instruction coming from anyone that I can remember. After a period of time sitting there, I realized that fact and just followed the clients from group to group to lunch to education and then left when I was supposed to leave. I did this for the first couple of days, and then, finally, people started "reluctantly" talking to me. I think some of them thought I was a client there for a while. I went to my counselor (he did not appear thrilled to have to "deal" with me), and he gave me minimal direction. My clinical supervisor told me that the "fending for yourself" I did the first week was a way to weed out some interns who would need too much direction. I was naïve, and I bought it. What I found out later on (I have taken on twenty-two interns over the past eleven years) is that people are so busy and inundated with paperwork, they don't have time to work with interns, and most don't want to. FC used the twelve-step program as their modality and had some grizzled old timers that were still on staff. "Grace" became my go-to person, and we would read the daily meditations together before we went to staffing in the morning. I was only able to intern four hours per day due to my 2:00 pm to 10:00 pm shift at Cronin. I did not have the luxury of ever not working, so I trudged through school methodically while working full-time jobs. I completed twenty hours per week until I started asking if I could come in and do some Saturdays. I had a forty-five-mile drive one way, so I spent ninety minutes driving, four hours interning, and then eight and a half hours working. This schedule kept me busy, obviously, but I was determined to get some semblance of a life back, no matter how many obstacles were in the way. I was just dialed in to the "newness" of it all. Little did I know that the accumulation of hours working with this population would exact a toll on me. A minimal amount of time was spent in my graduate courses talking about burnout and compassion fatigue, which is sad, as the career expectancy of an addiction counselor is three years.

The Cronin Home was the beginning of my work with chronic alcoholics and addicts, and it seemed to be a seamless transition. My job duties were to cook and serve forty-four residents, clean up the kitchen, distribute medications, count medications, do room searches, clean the building, UA residents, breathalyze them when they returned from being out in the community, and log anything of relevance in the logbook. You just couldn't ever give an inch with these folks, and you had to be on your "A" game. Then there was the internship, which had its learning moments as I learned the FC system of documentation. I was videotaped doing a three-hour group, did a bunch of assessments and treatment plans, and started to get to know the people who worked there. I was getting my first glimpse into the life of an addictions professional from an inpatient and a sober home perspective. These were great experiences for me. The Cronin Home was the best job I have ever had in my recovery, as I did not have to take the job home with me, and I felt that most of the residents appreciated me. It was a great experience, and I actually worked there for over three years (a good chunk of time for this restless wanderer).

As I was working evening shifts and only getting four or five hours per day at FC, I began to work some Saturdays, which allowed me to begin the process of working with families. This became a big part of my future curriculum and program. I loved the family education sessions with the parents and family members, and those were Saturdays from about eight to four. I had an amazing person to supervise me, and her name was "Jeanine." She was the family program counselor and basically took me under her wing and let me run three of these lengthy family sessions. She would give me very honest feedback, both good and bad. She didn't sugarcoat things, and she taught me when to push and when to back off, when to use the skill of empathy, and how to work with family systems. She was one of the best supervisors I have ever had. I learned more from her in the four months working with her than anyone else I have worked with, and her lessons stayed with me. My internship was trudging along, and then I was introduced to the drama and politics that run rampant in this industry. As I approached the halfway mark of my internship, I was applying for various jobs that would be posted on the internal site, and I finally moved up the ladder enough to get an interview. What followed was almost enough to push me over the edge.

"We are Rescinding Your Job"

I applied for a job at FC in October (no response), November (response but no job), and in December (scored interview). This particular job was a "float" position, which meant that I was to fill in for various counselors that used Personal Time Off (PTO), complete chemical health assessments, run education groups, etc. I interviewed twice and was officially offered the job on December 22nd 2010. I accepted the position, and was going to be able to be a paid intern for the last 440 hours of my internship. I put in my two weeks notice at Cronin and was given a date in early January to start. I thought I had arrived. I took my first long weekend (four total days) since leaving treatment three and a half years ago, and I remember going to a movie with my mother on the first of those four days (a Thursday). I was so happy and overcome with humility, and it felt good to feel this way. I had worked so hard these years, put in so much work, and tried to do it all with integrity. When I got home from the movie, I saw that FC had called and decided to call them the next day. It was the Human Resources department, and my PTSD kicked in before I even heard what was said. They rescinded my job offer with absolutely no remorse, stating that I had failed to include a misdemeanor theft on the application. I had included my felony DWI, the other four DWIs, my felony theft (now a misdemeanor), and my DACs (driving after cancellation). I certainly did not omit this on purpose. She stated they would be discussing my job hire on Monday, that I was not invited to this, and that they would be giving me a phone call to let me know what they decided. I was shocked and needless to say, my weekend was ruined since I would spend it obsessing over all of this. Monday came, and they called me to inform me that, indeed the job was rescinded, but I could still intern there since I was being "supervised." I "heard" later that the real reason for the rescinded job offer was due to the Mayo Clinic taking over the company on January 1st, 2011, and they did not want any felons working for Mayo. I don't know if this is true. So... the following Friday, I drove there, talked to my Clinical Supervisor, got all my documents signed off, and made the decision to walk away from my internship with 500 hours completed. I could not go back there after that. I was jobless and now looking for a site to complete my internship. I was devastated, demoralized, and felt shameful—these thoughts were eerily similar to the last years of my addiction. It was a hopeless feeling and one of the hardest days of my recovery. My criminal past was laid out for all to see once again.

Picking up the Pieces

I knew that Cronin would take me back, but my position was filled internally. The only position they had was a weekend overnight position on Fridays and Saturdays from 10:00 pm to 6:00 am. I took it. I was also hired back part-time at Dollar Tree and got about fifteen hours per week there. I was able to pick up shifts at Cronin sporadically for people wanting days off, and this helped me pay the bills. However, my world was turned upside down. I was resentful and bitter at how this all turned out, and although I have worked multiple fourth and fifth steps over the years, I continued to struggle with this for a period of time. I spent the next couple of months picking up shifts at Cronin, picking up as many shifts as I could at Dollar Tree, and restabilizing my emotional health. In late February, I started sending out some flyers to different treatment centers, looking for an opportunity. I remember four different visits to a halfway house in Rochester, but they had not had an intern before, and they were unable to pull the trigger. I looked into several outpatient programs and finally walked into one that would take me on. I was relieved and overcome with gratitude for this company. They did a background check, and I waited. Finally, on April 1st, 2011, my background check came back for this organization, which required me to do a "set aside," which is something the DHS requires if you have a criminal background. A "set aside" is a litany of documents you must provide to show you are "rehabilitated," which includes going back and answering questions about your arrests. The DHS needed "more time" to make a decision, but they did allow me to work with supervision. I began the second piece of my internship on April 11th, 2011. Over three months had passed since the debacle at FC, and I had put myself in a position once again to feel good about my future.

My First Counseling Job – The Fine Art of Redemption

I began the second phase of my 880-hour internship at an outpatient facility, and it was a "mom and pop" operation that employed a couple of my instructors at Winona State. They had a small "sprinkling" of staff and were known as a mental health center that did CD treatment. I started in the evening group with "B," and she ran group from 6:30 pm to 9:30 pm, three nights per week (Monday, Wednesday, Thursday). This worked well with my other jobs, and I started chipping away at my hours once again. I was eventually hired full-time at Cronin once again, and this time it was the 6:00 am to 2:00 pm shift. This allowed me to, once again, quit Dollar Tree and focus on forty hours at Cronin and twenty at the outpatient facility. I had officially "survived" the FC situation and felt like my current setup was better for me, without the drive, a slight raise at Cronin, and another counseling experience. It is funny how you get ideas in your head about what you want to do, and don't allow yourself to just let God be the Director. I love the quote I have heard often at AA meetings that goes, "I plan, God laughs." It was fitting for me on my journey. I thought FC was going to be my career and inpatient treatment, my forte. This was never going to work, but at the time, I couldn't see myself doing anything else. I had pigeonholed myself into a corner with expectations, and that is why I was so devastated (and fearful). This new place was another opportunity, and early on, I was very grateful for the opportunity. I hit the four-year mark of sobriety, was working with addicts (which was helping me), and I finished my internship in August of 2011, which was almost one year to the day when I started the 880 hours. I was the first student to finish the Winona State LADC certificate program, which was designed for people who already had bachelor's degrees in other helping professions. I put together my material for the Board of Behavioral Health and mailed it out at the end of the month. In the interim, the facility hired me as a part-time assessor, and paid me seventy-five dollars for each assessment done. I averaged twelve assessments per month, and I would come in and do them in the evening. The evening counselor quit at the end of October, and they offered me the night counselor position. I began in November, which meant I went to "on call" status at Cronin. I had achieved a major goal of mine four and a half years after getting sober, and that was to once again join the professional ranks in the helping professions. However, with that goal, came a price and it put a big, juicy target on my back, which was my addiction-based criminal past. Employers, licensing boards, and the DHS have been all too willing to tear the scab off my past, and I have had to relive it over and over again. This time it was the Board of Behavioral Health and Therapy—my licensing board.

My Meeting with the Board of Behavioral Health

When people make the decision to get sober, many don't think too far into the future, especially those who have a history of legal charges. I received a summons from the Board of Behavioral Health to come and meet with them on March 29, 2012. It took them five months to even get back to me after sending them my application, and then I had to wait another month to go and see them. Now, mind you, I had five life-time DWIs, a felony theft, one other theft, three DACs, and a damage to property ticket. I knew there were going to be questions, but the way this was handled was not how I envisioned it. I had to drive to Minneapolis on that Thursday for the afternoon meeting, and I arrived there with a lot of trepidation and fear. I had made a lot of progress in my life, but there was no guarantee they were going to allow me to be a professional in the field of addictions. Thoughts of relapse were dancing in my head, especially if things went sour. I had already planned it out, to be honest. The attendees at this meeting were the members of the Board, the assistant attorney general, and the administrative faction of the BBHT. I believe all together, there were twelve of them sitting there, and they began to ask me questions. Here was my favorite: "Can you tell me what the following numbers mean to you, Tim—25, 18, 16, 13, 12, 11, 10, 8?" I couldn't for the life of me figure this one out, so the answer was "no." "These are how many years ago, you committed a crime. Do you see a pattern? How can we be sure this pattern does not continue?" Fair question, just asked in a really strange way. I answered that all of those crimes were the result of my alcoholism—either directly or indirectly. I told them I was approaching five years of sobriety and was continuing to rebuild my life. After the rest of the questions, they sent me out to the hallway so they could talk about me. I felt like a ten-year -old being shamed by his "superiors." It was like getting a time-out. Were they getting off on this? I thought so. As I sat out there for about ten minutes, my relapse was set up. What a waste of the past five years, I thought to myself. "What kind of beer am I going to buy? Will the crack dealers still remember me?" They proceeded to call me back in and gave me the good news and the bad news. The good news was that they were going to allow me to be licensed as a LADC. The warmest relief washed over me. However, everything in my life seems to come with a price, and this time was no different. They fined me for each of the last six months that I did not have a valid license, as my internship was completed in August, and I was employed by the facility as a counselor or assessor since September. My co-workers had all written me letters of recommendation, and the proof of my operating without a license was apparent. "Don't you know the Code of Ethics, Mr. Volz? If you did, you would know it specifically states one cannot operate CD treatment without a license." These guys seemed to really be getting off on bludgeoning me. The fine was $295 multiplied by six months, or a cool $1770. They allowed me to make arrangements and told me that it would not appear on my LADC jacket if it was paid in full within six months. They bid me adieu, and I was on my way, excitement tempered by the fine and the verbal beat downs by the board members. They really made me feel like a criminal and not a person. It was demeaning and gross, and I felt like I was punished for being an alcoholic/addict. I paid a heavy price for my alcoholism, and no one can punish me as much as I punished myself. I understood there were going to be questions, but I did not think they would go after the jugular like they did, attempting to take away my humanity. I will never forget it, and it drives me today. I did get a chance to see this group again when attending an event for tiered licensing in Mankato in 2014, but they did not appear to even recognize me (or chose not to acknowledge me.) My criminal past has never relinquished its hold on me, and some people seem to take delight in trying to hold this over my head.

I got back to the facility, and of course, they were elated. They agreed to pay $700 of the fine, leaving me with the rest. It was paid on time, and to date, no marks have appeared on my license, although there have been multiple attempts to smear me and end my career, as you will hear about throughout the journey. I spent the next fifteen months at this facility, and I will give you a brief synopsis of my first year as a licensed counselor, including when a naïve counselor started to figure out the intricacies of counseling, and the craziness that lies bubbling beneath the surface.

My caseload at my employer became intense, and soon the room could barely house the horde of clients. My group grew to thirty-five clients (DHS states the maximum is sixteen), but I felt like I owed them and didn't complain (they damn sure didn't complain either, as I was the ultimate earner for them). I liked large groups, but they wore me down to a nub. I felt some pride in the size of the groups, but looking back, this also fed my ego, which was growing again. I ran Monday, Wednesday, and Thursday evening groups, facilitated the eight and twelve-hour DWI classes, completed two assessments per week, conducted as many individual sessions as I could, had five interns under my watch, and completed all the paperwork that a large caseload requires. It was a lot to ask of a person, and to this day, I do not understand why they put that kind of pressure on me my first year. I was also working about one shift per week at Cronin Home. This meant I was leaving the house at 7:30 am, getting home around 10:00 pm, and my weekly hours usually averaged seventy-five to eighty. Looking at this today, it is easy to see how I slowly started to reach compassion fatigue and then burnout. The game changer for me in my first two years of counseling was the opioid crisis and how that created a huge ripple effect in the community. There was a well-publicized overdose death in 2012 that was strewn all over the papers and the news, and at the funeral, one of my clients showed up and was actually clean!! The "faded out" mourners asked him how he did it, and he told them he was attending a longer-term outpatient treatment program, and my phone just blew up. I had fifteen to twenty heroin addicts calling for assessments within the first two weeks after the funeral, and they all wanted to come to treatment together. After about two months, I knew they needed their own group, as they felt they were not understood by the alcoholics and stimulant addicts in group, and they felt stigmatized. I started running this new group once per week but soon realized this group needed three nights per week, so one of the owners started running my old group, and I took on the heroin population. It was a beast. I did not enjoy this population very much at all, as heroin addiction is something that cannot be treated like traditional outpatient treatment. The level of deceit and relapse is over the top compared to other populations, and you also had the "overdose dilemma" to deal with. No one wants to see a heroin addict die on their watch. This population needs medication, therapy, groups where there is long-term accountability with urine screens, and probably some contingency management at first. At some point, they need a medication taper as well. The biggest problem, however, was that most outpatient treatment facilities where I lived wouldn't even take someone in their program if they were on Suboxone or Methadone. I changed that; I took them (90 mg. max for methadone), and it made a big difference. This difficult population started to take its toll on me after some time, and I became fatigued and a bit anguished. I then started to look at the facility I worked at much closer and started to see some "patterns" in our Monday morning clinical meetings.

Our Monday morning clinical meetings were absolutely useless, and they would basically be about the same each week. The owners would tell the team at some point that their facility was "the best-kept secret in town." At some point, they would bash two or three of their competitors, and it became obvious that they were insecure as a facility. The owners would also make remarks like, "We take the toughest clients in the city, and no one else takes them." This "clinical" meeting was always just a reason for the owners to talk about how they work eighty hours per week, how they took out loans to pay their employees when times were tough, how other programs were inadequate, and why. Some of the interns I worked with (did I mention that I had FIVE under my watch in my first year of counseling) expressed some discomfort in hearing them "preach" in the mornings. I took off my "rose-tinted" glasses and started to view this organization with a different lens. There appeared to be a lack of professionalism, but some of their long-term employees just bought right into it, it seemed.

The Final Days and a Move

I had been there almost two years in March of 2013 and thought I would set up an appointment to meet with the owners about a potential raise. I was putting in the hours, had started a new group, and had admitted over a hundred clients in my first year. I estimated I had brought in about $500,000 in this past year (maybe a lot more), as the owners now had the luxury to rent an adjoining building to double their space in order to hire more counselors. The billing person let me know that my earnings were a big reason why. So... I asked for a raise and advocated for myself. I was getting paid eighteen dollars per hour for thirty-five hours per week (working seventy), and I wanted a five-dollar raise. In other words, I was basically getting paid nine dollars per hour, which is the same I made while serving customers at the meat counter. They looked appalled at this and got defensive. One of the owners stated, "This company is not called 'Timpower'". He was vehement in stating that no other company would ever consider hiring me due to my past criminal record. They basically debased me and offered me two dollars per hour. I accepted this but walked out of there knowing what they thought of me as a person. When I got home after my twelve-hour Monday, there was a flyer in the mailbox from the Adolescent Treatment Center in Winnebago, MN. I thought, *the irony of that.* I had no idea where Winnebago was, but I arranged an interview. . .because "no one would hire me." That statement stuck in my craw for a long time, and it was not the first time they had let everyone know that they had "taken a chance on me when no one else would." The first time was at their annual Christmas party, in front of a lot of people. *They were letting me know my place*, I thought. All of this really came to a head the day of that meeting, and I realized that there was no future for me there.

I took my first day off work since I began eighteen months earlier and wended my way to Winnebago. The interview went well, and the facility was new and fresh. Winnebago was a small town in Faribault County, which was very small in county size, with about 33,000 souls. They did not get a lot of candidates to apply because of the location, but they liked me and told me they would be in touch. They called me a week later and offered me the job, which was to start the first outpatient adolescent program in Faribault County, which seemed daunting. I accepted it and put in a one-month notice immediately. I went back there, filled out the application, did the background check and signed the contract. When I came back to work (I had now taken two days off work in eighteen months), there was a nice passive-aggressive email from one of the owners, which was demeaning, stating I was doing this wrong, doing that wrong, and "people are not going to be upset when you leave." It was a scathing and biting email, but I let this go; I was ready to move on. I got all my paperwork done, moved clients through the program if they were ready, and thinned down my opiate group. They hired a new counselor, and it appeared everyone was handling the transition. It was awkward and uncomfortable at times, but I got the sense that all parties involved were handling this with professionalism and courtesy. I vividly remember going back to my place of employment with my U-Haul full of stuff and thanking them for the opportunity they gave me right before moving the majority of my things to Winnebago. It was the last place I went before hitting the road. I was acting with a lot of integrity and was letting them know that I appreciated them, despite the way I was talked to and treated the last month I was there. Recovery has taught me a lot about integrity and doing the right things (despite what others think). It is one of my four core values today. I was oblivious to the "hammer" that was about to be dropped on me, and it created one of the biggest resentments I have ever had to overcome. As a matter of fact, it affected me to the core daily for about five months.

Leaving for the Wild West (of Minnesota)

I found a small home to rent in Winnebago, and my landlord in Rochester allowed me to stay there for $300 per month, so I could come back to Rochester on weekends. I was to live in "Bago" Monday through Friday and come back Friday night and stay until early Monday. I knew this wasn't going to last, but it bought me some time to see if I liked the job, the community, and the move. I liked all three and eventually just moved over to Winnebago. It was on to working with adolescents. I was to build an outpatient treatment program at ATCW and began this in the summer of 2013. It was a slow go, and in the interim, I did some work in the inpatient unit, such as running some groups. I ran my first outpatient group at the end of June when I was able to get my first five clients. I have to admit, working with adolescents in Faribault County was a big career move from adults, but I gave it a chance. Over the course of that summer, I was able to build this outpatient program in rural Minnesota to capacity with sixteen clients. I couldn't believe it!! I vividly remember sitting in the group room one evening in September and looking around the room, counting sixteen people. There were two girls sitting in one corner of the room with nose rings, staring at me, and I remember thinking, *Is this what I signed up for?* The program was growing, and it was my job to market it as well. I went to several schools in the county, met with human services people at Faribault County and showed up at meetings and committees. I was making a name for myself and familiarizing myself with the community and the different schools in the area. I continued with outpatient through the end of the year but eventually moved to inpatient programming, as several counselors either quit or were fired. I was working with an intern, and she took over the outpatient programming, although I was still able to oversee it. I enjoyed the jump to inpatient treatment and was enjoying the transition to living in a small town. I found a great AA meeting in town called the "Shivering Denizens," and it was a nice Friday night two-hour, open meeting. It became my new home group. I also found a good meeting in Mankato and began to get acclimated into the recovery community. This was very important for me, as I moved the rest of my belongings to Winnebago in November and made it official. I was now living exclusively in Bago and had been looking to purchase a house. As the year flipped to 2014, I was becoming settled and satisfied with my decision to make a geographical change.

The Unfounded Grievance and
the Reality of this "Profession"

I found a beautiful three-bedroom home and purchased it in January 2014. I moved in at the end of January, and I was feeling like my life was becoming full. I never envisioned seven years ago that I would be buying a home, living in a "still foreign" area, and not have the desire to drink or do drugs. I felt like I had a life, and I had time for trips back to Rochester. I found a sponsor in Mankato, started working the steps again and had a good life balance. Dare say I was happy? I really think I felt some joy and happiness for the first time in a long time. It was fleeting. A casual Friday stroll to the mailbox on Friday, February 28th, was all it took, and all the anxiety, fear, anger, and hatred came back to me in a huge ball of angst. The owners of my previous place of employment had filed a grievance against me with the Board of Behavioral Health and Therapy for the following: (1) Stating that I would hold client's money for them and distribute it when they needed it (as a form of relapse prevention), and (2) asking to borrow $5000 from a client for help in purchasing a house. I read the letter over and over again, not believing they had done this to me. Both of these accusations were things I had not allegedly done but things I allegedly said. I was stunned. I took the time to flesh out a letter to the board, explaining that I understand the Code of Ethics and that these charges are categorically false. I sent it back and began to worry, and then worry some more. I had come so far, but when you have a past like mine, it is easy to catastrophize. That is exactly what I did. It was exhausting and mentally fatiguing. Was my past being used against me? Why would they do this? I had just bought my first house. Am I going to lose my career? It was hard not to obsess over this. This is exactly what they wanted when they sent this through the mail. I sent the letter back on March 3rd, and then I heard absolutely nothing for months. I called the BBHT and asked what the holdup was. I finally received a letter in mid-July stating that the case was closed due to no proof of either accusation. Of course, they had no proof—these were things that allegedly someone said that I SAID—not that I actually did. It was a horrible thing to do by reported Christians. To top it all off, the reason it took so long to receive the letter was that the board sent the letter to my old address (the wrong address), even though I changed my address with the board (required) the previous May when I changed job locations. I sat and worried daily for two months because the board sent their "decision" to the wrong address. This whole thing was a complete shit show, and some old PTSD crept in during those months, which was due to my past consequences. It was very traumatic, and the experiences I went through had shown me that this needed to be opened up and talked about, then discarded. What was born out of these despicable actions by the owners of a treatment center was a resentment that festered and lingered until 2019. Righteous anger is a bitch. Rest assured, my caution level went way up, and it was only through some of the good people I encountered at ATCW that I stayed in the field of counseling after that. I didn't know at the time that my future would hold an opportunity to chat with my former employers, but I am grateful for that opportunity. I want to tell you that the years I spent taking jobs of humility, biking everywhere, and turning my life around were never taken into consideration by these people before trying to end my career. They were looking to target someone who decided to leave their company. I can also tell you that there were numerous ethical violations that were facilitated by the owners, including storing medications for clients, allowing thirty-plus people in my group, having interns bill for sessions and the owner flashing his gun to his staff every chance he got. I just never felt I had the ill will stored in me to do that to someone else. It is sad to me that there are people who would attack someone's character through a grievance when they are a hundred miles away, had moved on, and made their business a lot of money. This affected me deeply, including my trust level with professionals, and it hardened me a little as well. This is what I signed up for when I made the decision to help people for a career? I never forgot that feeling, and it changed my view of the treatment profession.

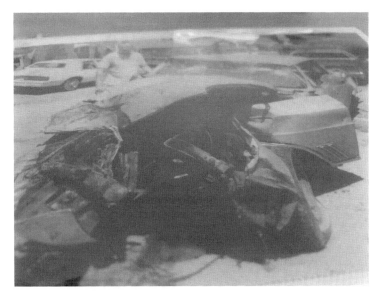

1987 - DWI #1

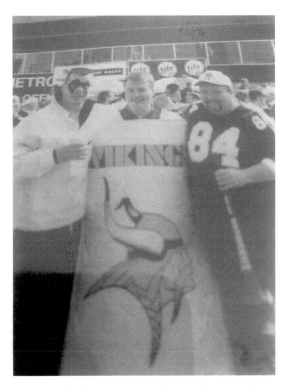

Alcohol and Viking games were fixtures of my using days.

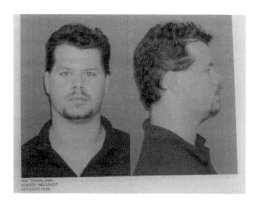

Booking photo #1

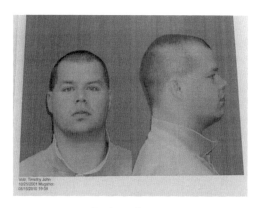

Booking photo #2

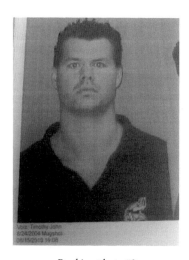

Booking photo #3

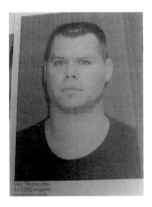

Booking photo #4

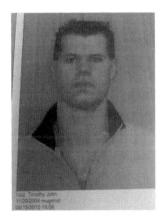

Booking photo #5

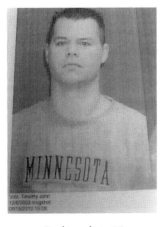

Booking photo #6

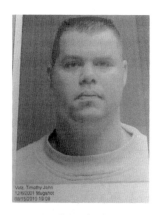

Booking photo #7

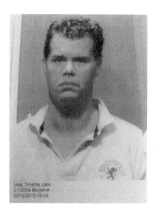

Booking photo #8

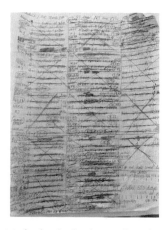

My final jail calendar in all its glory

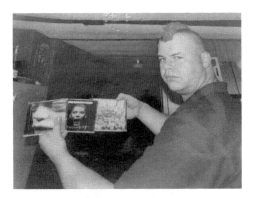

2001 – Ready for Rammstein

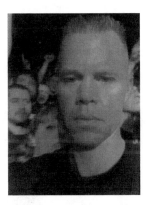

Front row, sweaty, and sober at Amon Amarth

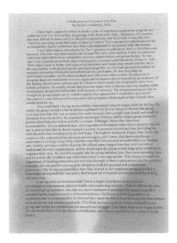

The day I knew long-term IOP would work

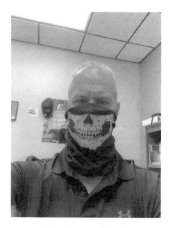

IOP in 2020 with masks

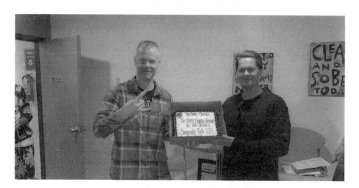

Coining out Robb – RIP man

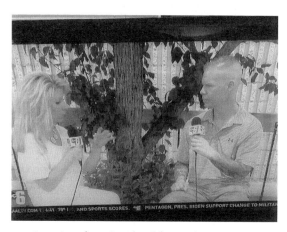

Interview about Covid and face-to-face treatment

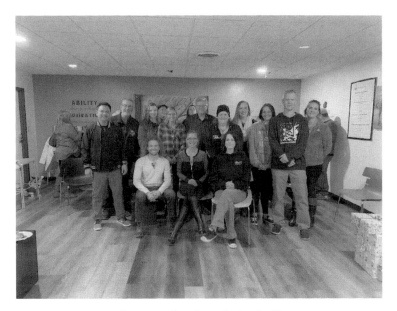

One-year sober clients during Covid

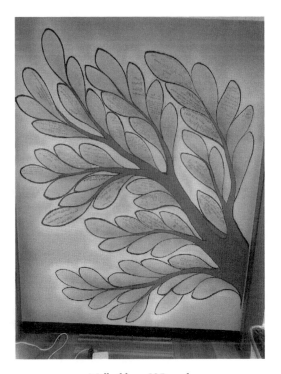

Wall of fame IOP grads

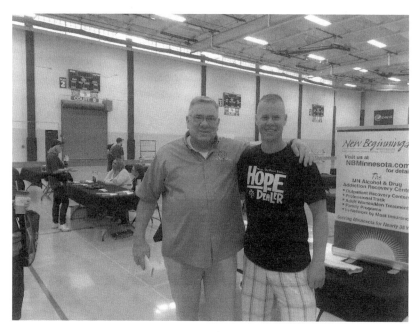

Recovery man John Shinholser

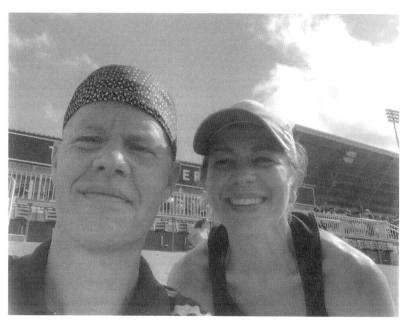

With Molly in Fort Myers, FL

Beginning My Master's Program
and the Drug Court Opportunity

I officially began my master's program in May of 2014 and started taking classes through Walden University. This decision was something that picked up steam when I moved to a small town where I had the time to do the schoolwork. This program was completely online, other than two residencies taken over the course of the program. Living in a small town was the perfect opportunity to begin this program, but little did I know the incredible amount of sacrifice it would take. I was excited to be back in school, and I wanted to remain teachable and learn more about the mental health component. It was 105 credits, and it turned into a five-year grind (seven if you count the two years of clinical supervision). I was now a forty-six-year-old student and mature enough in my sobriety to utilize the grit and mental toughness it takes to get through a program while working full-time and working a recovery program. This business did take its toll, though. My self-care suffered, and my life passions were not being nurtured. School took up every one of my Saturdays for five years straight (more on that later). I started churning out the coursework and APA-style papers and became a writing machine. I had just completed my first two courses when I received a phone call from two men who owned an outpatient treatment program in Mankato/St. Peter. They were losing their Nicollet Drug Court treatment counselor and needed someone to come in and work with this population. They had heard "good things" about me and wanted to interview me. At this time, I was working in the inpatient part of ATCW, and although I liked the job, I had found that my preference was to work with adults. I went to two interviews, and after the second interview, I accepted the offer and took the job. I started in September of 2014. Working with drug court was something I had always wanted to do, and although the drive from Winnebago was forty-five miles (ninety round trip), I relished the opportunity to continue to grow as a counselor. It was hard to put in my notice, and my supervisor was very sad (and actually got emotional before apologizing), which was the exact opposite reaction I got from my previous employer. We left on great terms, which turned out to be a good thing, as my time at this facility was not over by any means. It also somewhat restored my faith in this field, as it had been trampled on by the experiences I had during my internship and first job. Naomi remains a good friend to this day!

The Year of Working with Two
Drug Courts Simultaneously

Working in St. Peter began with meeting the Drug Court team, including the judge, drug court coordinator, probation officers, jailers, attorneys, and drug task force detectives. The judge asked me a simple question right off the bat, which was, "Have you ever been to jail before?" I replied, "Which time?" She said, "Good." At that juncture of the interview, I knew that this was going to be a different experience than in the past. She was looking not only for a counseling professional but someone with whom the participants could relate and respect. The St. Peter location was in the bowels of a large apartment building—Park Row apartments. It was an old, musty heap, and the day I started, I went down to my office, and the only other employee (mental health therapist) working in the office came up, shook my hand, and told me she had just resigned this morning and had put in her notice. This was a red flag right off the bat, but I was not interested in the "why's" at that time. I had to learn a lot of new stuff. I was back to working with adults, but this time was a little different, with the addition of drug court responsibilities. My group started with six participants, but in the next three months, I started taking people other than drug court participants into programming, and I was up to twenty clients. This number ballooned to thirty when the company contracted with Le Seuer County Drug Court in January of 2015, and I began my travels to Le Center to head up the treatment part of that team. My weekly schedule included two drug court appearances, running three groups, all the paperwork a large caseload requires, assessments, and individual sessions. It was about 60 hours per week.

I also drove ninety miles per day, was taking master's level classes, and was the only staff member working in the office most days. The schedule was grueling, but I was satisfied at first, as this was a population that appealed to me.

I will tell you that working with drug court clients can be exhausting. They are needy and have layers and layers to unpeel. Working with one county drug court is a challenge, but working with two is just plain ridiculous. Le Seuer County was a pilot drug court, so there were mandatory trainings and a lot to unpack. I was not getting any help (a common theme in this field), and to be honest, I was scared to work with female drug court participants one-on-one as I was the only counselor in the office. It was not long before I started to burn out, especially around April, when the Le Sueur County hit about ten participants. It was too much driving, too many clients, and too much paperwork. I made the decision to speak my mind and advocate for myself getting some help, as the facility psychologist started coming once per week to do therapy, and he couldn't believe my caseload. He told me that this caseload is not sustainable and went back and reported to his bosses that "Tim needs some help." The owners responded by sending an email to everyone in the organization, stating that I had been "complaining" about my workload. No one came to see me to communicate with me. This was just a long email that did not do anything but point fingers. It took the company two months to send anyone to help, and by then, I was outraged and damaged. The organization I worked for had been the treatment provider for Drug Court for many years, and I started talking to members of the team (including the judge) about switching to another provider. They were on board with keeping me if I moved to another organization, and the judge even made some inquiries. However, the owners sensed something was adrift and set up a meeting during Drug Court, and once again, I was taking the fall for being the "bad guy." The target once again fell squarely on my back. The owners of the company did not address the fact that I was the sole treatment provider for two drug courts, which both had twelve to fourteen clients at the time. They talked about me as if I weren't even in the room, calling me "controversial" and other denigrating words. The Drug Court team stayed relatively quiet, and it was during this time at this staffing, sitting there getting belittled, that I decided I was done there. I left the meeting and had a conversation with a co-worker that I trusted within the agency, venting a little, and he went directly to the owners with this. There was nothing that was sacred. I made the decision to go back to work at my old employer with adolescents (who were elated to have me back) and put in my notice that day. They immediately sent a counselor to come and take my spot, telling me they accepted my resignation and to immediately leave, with no closure with clients. They had the gall to send my "friend," who followed me from the adolescent treatment center to this company, to take my spot. She showed up and watched me pack my belongings and walk away. It was surreal. Of course, the drama did not simply end there. They had to attempted to sully my name (the new counselor did, too), and tried to take down a drug court team member and social worker I had befriended who worked for the county. This further divided my loyalty to the profession, as the schisms that developed over the course of helping difficult clients were so unprofessional and unbelievable (ego is the reason). The owners accused my social worker friend of sleeping with me and of inappropriate relations during work hours. An intern told them she would come over, and we would staff clients with the door closed—this was true. He also told them he could hear laughing in the office and accused us of having a relationship. They threw my friend under the bus and effectively tried to get her fired. None of it was true, of course, and I was left completely out of the situation, but my friend was accosted and humiliated. She ultimately was exonerated of any wrongdoing. The Drug Court team also eventually changed treatment providers, and the two owners sold their company. However, the administrators in charge of these programs left emotional scars on people that take time to heal. This leads me to one of the most important lessons that I have learned by watching other professionals in the CD field: Don't stop working a strong recovery program—we never "arrive." This is one of the most important lessons I will try to impress upon the new counselor who is in recovery—don't stop working your recovery program.

I have seen this happen too many times to count, and this is an invaluable lesson that I have learned about the counselor in recovery. Many people get sober and set out to become counselors in the state of Minnesota. They make it ridiculously easy with this asinine "2+2 program," which allows students to become addictions counselors with an associate's degree, provided they complete an 880-hour internship. What I have seen happen ad nauseam, is that they reach their goal of becoming a counselor, and they forget where they came from. They, in effect, stop working their own program and utilize their counseling platform as a place to work their own recovery. This is a huge mistake, and it usually leads to client harm.

This also leads to counselors stagnating and burning out. Continuous growth should be the motto, and I am eternally grateful that I continue to go to meetings, work with a sponsor, utilize clinical supervision outside the agency where I work, and work a comprehensive, holistic program as well, with physical health and music being HUGE parts of my regimen (more on that in the last section of the book).

At this time in my relatively new career, I had worked at three places, and two of them felt very unhealthy. The place that didn't was run by some-one not in "recovery," and she was an amazing director. I had resentments, and I had lost some trust in the field of counseling, so I had to double down on my own program, which meant reworking the steps with my sponsor "Vince." This saved my bacon and gave me a different, newer recovery per-spective. The importance of working a strong recovery program in the field of addictions is paramount, or one can find themselves bagging groceries in no time. Anyway, I digress. . .back to the adolescent treatment center for my second stint.

Adolescent Treatment Center – Second Stint

My second trip back to the adolescent treatment center proved to be nothing more than a job, as everything had changed. The counseling assistants, or CD technicians, had become bullies since I left and had started to turn against the counselors. It reminded me of the William White book, *The Incestuous Workplace*. To paraphrase, White talks about "surviving when finding oneself in destructive work environments." My old program director put in her notice about two months after I got back (I didn't blame her), and she promoted a counselor to her spot that had been loyal to the agency for about five years. I totally understood the move, as it was done out of respect for someone who had paid their dues. However, I also knew that the CD techs would feast on her, as she was a little soft. I was not going to be stuck in a situation where the CD techs were turning clients against their counselors, so I decided to make this a short stay. Now, this made it three out of four agencies I had worked at where sickness had permeated from the inside out. Clients could see it and feel the tension. I felt stuck and reached out to an agency I admired and had an interview with them at the end of the year. I made the decision to take the "satellite job" in St. Peter and started in early April of 2016. This facility allowed me to be myself, and I had known a lot of professionals through my last job in St. Peter, so it was a great fit. It was also where I introduced my curriculum for a long-term outpatient treatment program, which was something that I started to develop when I worked for Drug Court in 2014. This program is the only one that I know of that is twelve to eighteen months in length, with witnessed UA accountability and 500 hours of programming. This new facility is where I started the program and planted the seed.

St Peter Part II – "New Beginnings"—Literally

My second counseling job in St. Peter was a great fit, and this was a satellite office for the "mothership" in Waverly, which was their inpatient facility. I loved the location, the setup, and my experience working in another satellite office made this opportunity an easy transition. I took over an evening group that had about ten people, and within three months, it was overflowing and full. The night counselor went to days, and we had an intern there—that was all.

I enjoyed the autonomy, and our clinical supervisor was a great person who came down once per month and met with us, and offered up Zoom for the rest of the month. I started to dabble in research about long-term outpatient care and found little on the specifics but a lot on the benefits of retention in treatment. Drug Courts utilize a period of 225-250 treatment hours, and I thought that worked great with my clients previously. I began piecing together topics for different modules to put together enough material for one year. It was a labor of love, as I had four different work experiences to draw from and my twenty-two years of active use. How do I keep people invested and interested for that long of a period of time? It had to be interesting, educational, and insightful. I decided that I was not going to incorporate any movies or Ted Talks or drawing time (or any other filler) and make it strictly group talk therapy. I liked the results, and I could feel clients buying into long-term, as many had been in treatment ten or more times in the past. This was the place where I was able to practice and introduce my curriculum to clients, as I had the independence to run the evening program as I wished. The group started to grow immediately, and pretty soon, I was in a similar spot as in other places I worked. I was figuring out that with the education, life experience, consequences from using and drinking, and a quirky, dark sense of humor, I was able to build rapport with people in a unique way. People bought into what I was saying as I continued to work a recovery program of my own.

They listened because they knew I had been there. They respected me, and because of that, I could be hard on them at times. Although I had a criminal past, I started to really believe for the first time that I was an asset to employers. I still questioned inside if I was a good man, because of my past and the damage that was done by my drinking and drug use. I had been led to working with others as a passion, and started to grow an inner confidence and self-worth that matched my outside. My identity was starting to be established as someone who helped and mentored others. I was also building my resume by working at different facilities and watching for similarities and differences. I really liked this job and felt like the organization was invested in their people. I was happy there and was starting to feel like I could stay at this place for a while until I received a call one day from an old acquaintance back in Rochester who was looking to start an IOP for her Recovery Community Organization. She got me thinking about running my own program with complete autonomy. I questioned this as I made my way back to Rochester one weekend, representing my current facility at a recovery walk to benefit the RCO. It was in September of 2016 when I was finally able to meet face-to-face with the people responsible for trying to end my career.

Facing What Consumed Me

I told my current organization that I would "man" a table for the recovery walk in Rochester with pamphlets and information about their organization. I was planning on walking in it anyway. That Saturday morning was interesting, to say the least. I got to Rochester and walked into the field house, bringing a large sign, boxes of pamphlets, and some small giveaways with the company logo on them. I had had several conversations with The RCO about starting her treatment program, but I had not fully committed yet. What happened that day pushed me to take the position, although for the wrong reason. I allowed my character defects of pride and resentment to get in the way, although it has taught me a lot about my recovery then and my recovery now.

As soon as I walked into the building, the "grievance filers" must have known I was going to be present, as one of them immediately walked up to me and stated, "Can we just get along?" I proceeded to have a fifteen-minute conversation with him. Let me preface this by saying that this guy owns a treatment facility, is an alleged Christian, and is part of another organization that does compassion counseling (whatever that is). I let him know that I didn't appreciate the grievance filing and that it had been squashed by the Board of Behavioral Health. He stated he was "told by MARRCH" (Minnesota Association of Resources for Recovery and Chemical Health) that he had to file this. However, this was later refuted by three MARRCH members, who stated that they remember this guy talking to them about this, and they told him, if it bothered him that much, to give me a call. This guy just lied right to my face, and I told him as much. He then asked me if I was coming back to Rochester and that "it would be so great for the recovery community to have you back." Deep down inside, he was absolutely horrified that I was going to be coming back. It repulses me to think about that conversation, as he works with vulnerable clients, and just lied to my face. I walked away from that conversation feeling pity for that organization and anger that he tried so hard to paint a picture of himself as a good man when he actually tried to end my career with lies. Other than that, the day was awesome, and I walked away from this event having made my decision to come back to Rochester. I had some slight trepidation about coming back, but this was a career move and a chance to apply my curriculum and begin my own program of long-term intensive outpatient treatment. It was still a few months off, but I began preparing.

Making the Jump Back "Home"

It was hard to leave St. Peter because I would miss the independence, the clients (always the clients), and the people who worked there. It was an enjoyable year there, but I felt like I was ready for this new challenge, and I had a yearning to put my stamp on a treatment program. I started my new job in Rochester in January of 2017 on a part-time basis. Our outpatient license was handed out in late 2016, and I made the drive to Rochester most Fridays to do assessments and try to get a jump on building a group. My first official full-time day there was March 13th, and one week later, I had my first group, back in Rochester as a Treatment Director and primary counselor. I attended the CD consortium, which was a meeting for treatment providers, probation officers, and child protection workers, and I spoke to market the new program. I walked out of that meeting with a feeling that some were happy to have me back, and some would have been just fine if I never came back to Rochester. By July, I had thirty people in the program, and I was running full bore. It exploded. I got into Olmsted County drug court as a treatment provider, but this was not like the other two drug courts. Treatment clients were allowed to go to several different programs because of the number of participants. I felt like the drug court team was so much different than the other two drug courts. The treatment providers certainly did not carry the same weight as they did at the other two drug courts I had worked with. When I went to drug court trainings "Helen" would always say that the treatment professionals saw the client more than anyone, so they knew the client better than anyone. I had to bite my tongue many times, and other times I couldn't and spoke my truth.

I had some business back in Winnebago to take care of, like selling my house. This took some time, so in the interim, I stayed at my girlfriend Molly's home for two days, my mom's place for two days, and then went back to my home on weekends. I did my schoolwork at work during the week, and then wrote my papers and did my counseling videotapings for school on weekends. I attended my meetings, but at this point in my recovery, I did not have a sponsor anymore. I was attending a weekly meeting in Mankato, but my new job was keeping me very busy, and I was still in school. I was slowly falling out of recovery and into "just not drinking or using." I started to become irritable, and being back in Rochester was bittersweet. Some people were very happy for me, but several treatment providers were not, and the old jealousy game came back in full force.

Having the self-awareness to see that I needed to add more to my "recovery plate" is the result of daily deposits made over the years of recovery. That means I can make a withdrawal from my "recovery bank" when things get difficult. Physical exercise was something that has always been paramount to my recovery, as well as attending AA meetings, morning writing, prayer, and enjoying recovery fellowship. With my new job, new stressors, and being back in Rochester, I needed to embrace something new. I needed the guidance of a new sponsor, as well as a clinical supervisor, another gym membership, and a mentor. I found three different individuals to cover those roles, and it has made a big difference for me in my life. I found a gym two blocks from my job. I also found a church to attend, and that has been a huge factor in my spiritual growth. Without adding these assets and having the self-awareness to do that, I would have had a hard time with this transition. I loved my home and the quiet calmness of a small, rural town. Coming back to Rochester was something I needed to be talked into and at times, regretted deeply.

I quickly found out that not much had changed in four years of my being gone. I also found out that the person running this facility had acquired a reputation amongst some professionals in this city. She was an intern at the facility I had worked at previously in Rochester, and I also knew her from recovery meetings. There had been some accusations against one of her children, and they found some suspicious money at her home. Nothing came of it, but it was in the paper, and this created a small stain on the program I was starting. This made it awkward at times, especially when I made the decision to join the drug court team. There were other stressors as well. One of the attorneys on the drug court team had represented me back in 2004, and another one was a prosecuting attorney who tried to send me to prison two times. There was just a lot of stress on me, from starting a shiny new treatment program to facing the past again to working with someone that I respected but that others didn't. The reasons for leaving Rochester were soon back in full force, and this made things difficult at times.

We were audited by the Department of Human Services (DHS) in October, about six months after I started. This is normally done about every three years, but for new programs, they like to come in and look through random charts and employee files to ensure there is Rule 31 (now 245G) compliance. They had not let me know they were coming, and they showed up on a Thursday. I had drug court that day, and upon returning, I found out that two agencies in town had filed grievances with the DHS about me and the program. The three separate grievances filed stated that I had too many people in my groups (you could only average sixteen people per group), that I had given a client a sobriety medallion at an AA meeting and broke his confidentiality, and that I was "unprofessional." Some examples I was accused of included swearing, trying to steal clients from other programs, dressing inappropriately (you cannot make this up), and other forms of alleged "treachery." The other claim was based on an owner from another agency who would drive by the treatment center when there were group breaks and count the people outside smoking cigarettes. He used this as the basis of his grievance. I believe it was the same one who filed a grievance against me before, but cannot be sure. I was just absolutely floored that I was, once again, going to have to convince a board that I had not done anything to warrant any punitive sanctions. I explained myself to the DHS faction that had invaded my office space and told them I had not been to a meeting in Rochester where they gave out coins since 2012. I never tried to steal clients from other programs; rather, clients from other programs wanted to come to my group. They surprised me when stating that they had already talked to three of my current clients and "they all love you, Tim. They stated that you were professional in all your actions and the way you handle your groups." I once again was targeted six months into returning back to the "Med City." Nothing happened out of this, except I did get cited for averaging nineteen clients in the month of July. They were satisfied that the rest was untrue. These nameless people can just file grievance after grievance and can remain anonymous. However, it did not take much for me to figure out who the culprits were. I wonder why these people feel so threatened by my presence. I have talked to a few professionals that I trust, and they say it is jealousy. I don't know about that, but if they knew what I have to go through every time I change jobs in the addiction counseling field, they might rethink their angst. They are "jealous" of someone who still has to do a "Set Aside" with DHS every time he changes jobs for a Felony DUI from May of 2004. Trust me; they don't want to have to deal with that nuisance every time a job gets changed. I have had many doors closed on me due to my legal situation, including teaching and coaching jobs. More on "Set Asides" later.

2018 – Persistence and My Master's Degree…
and Another Job Change

I sold my house in January of 2018, and what a relief that was. I ended up finding a mobile home out in the country to rent in October of 2017 and moved all my stuff in there in January. College raged on, and now I was in my fifth year. I completed my last residency in Georgia at the end of 2017, and now I was preparing for another internship—nine months' worth. I was also required to take two family courses to ensure licensing, and these were cobbled into my schedule along with full-time employment and my internship. Up to this point, I had "ground" through the Walden University coursework one class at a time, starting in May of 2014. I was to end up with 105 credits for my master's, and I was down to three-quarters of interning and two family-based courses. There was a light at the end of the tunnel. I wrote roughly 250 APA-style papers over this time, as Walden was almost exclusively an online school (other than two one-week residencies). I was very tired of school, as I had spent almost seven of my eleven years of sobriety up to this point in college. I also sacrificed a lot of self-care during these years of school, as I could not get a lot of schoolwork done during the week, so my papers and discussion board responses were smashed into my weekends. One thing I will never forget about getting my master's degree is sitting at my kitchen table on a Saturday morning, looking outside at a gorgeous day, and knowing I had to sacrifice a round of golf to sit inside and hammer out a ten-page APA-style paper. This is where self-discipline and mental toughness came into play. These two learned skills are a big part of my recovery today and looking back now; I don't know if I would do this all over again. I was relentless about getting my master's degree. Now I had to look for a place to complete my internship. I had collaborated with a therapist when going through the Child Protection system with a mutual client, and I called and asked her if I could intern there. She asked the owner of the facility and BOOM. . .I began my internship in May at a mental health facility called Blue Stem. This facility worked with both adolescents and adults, providing mental health therapy, including medication management. It was a perfect fit for me, as I wanted to work in a place where I could learn a lot and work with professionals in the mental health field. I had reconfigured my balance once again, as I had 750 hours to complete in three quarters. This place allowed me to learn so much, and it was a great decision and choice.

As far as my place of employment, it was getting to be a burden. When I started, there were only three people working there, and everyone had their space. I was able to get the program started, and my name was back out in the community. My group filled up fast, and this created a lot of paperwork. I began on the drug court team, and soon had between nine and eleven participants in my group. At the end of 2017 into 2018, the founder wrote a grant, and she received grant money to begin training Peer Recovery Coaches. She hired one and eventually, hired six. I had also hired a counselor to help with the treatment overflow. The place started to become chaotic, and there was no organizational flow with the peer coaches. Boundaries were being crossed, and no one understood what the code of ethics was all about. There were a bunch of coaches in early recovery running around, and I began to be disgusted with the craziness and chaos. Just think of a bunch of people between one and three years sober, running around with unchecked ADHD. It was a mess. I reached out to someone at another facility, interviewed, and was offered a position. This position came with a decrease in pay, but it was a co-occurring facility, and there appeared to be a lot of support there. I put in my notice in July and started there on August 16th, 2018. I brought every one of my clients with me, which might sound crass, but it was their choice. It caused consternation, of course, but I moved back to Rochester to begin a treatment program, so this facility could be self-sustaining. So…twenty-five clients and I made the pilgrimage across town to another treatment center. That had not been done before, and of course, some people in the professional community had a lot to say about that. I left the place and someone new came in and tried to run the program I started.

Another New Gig and
My Mental Health Internship

I started my mental health internship at the end of May of 2018 at Blue Stem. Two months later, I was working at a new facility (number seven) and admitting twenty-five clients who left my old facility and followed me to the new place. This was a larger company, with a campus on the outskirts of Rochester and a smaller building downtown. The person I reached out to had been working there for years, and right before I was hired, she retired. I had known her for years and trusted her, so this changed things, as I felt like my "go-to person" was gone. I started at the campus, but it became apparent, very quickly, that the people in human resources and myself were going to butt heads. They appeared to actually run the show out there—not the program directors and supervisors. They were penny pinchers, and not one single iota was given away. They had five or six SUD programs, from a harm reduction program to a co-occurring program to a program for first-time treatment participants. They were all basically the same, with countless videos and Ted Talks to watch. They wanted to name my program "Sustaining Recovery" due to its length. Now, if I was an employer and my new employee marched twenty-five brand new clients into the facility, I would be elated. This would also create some clients for the therapists to pick up as well. Unfortunately, the HR personnel made this a living hell for my people. They told me the clients could not start for two weeks while the insurance was being processed (it takes two days, which I knew from doing this at my previous place). If someone owed a co-pay of fifteen dollars, they would not let them come to group until that was paid. They were given little laminated squares when they walked in the door that stated "ok" or "Check with me." This meant that they owed money and would not be able to come to group until they forked over the cash. Now, everyone knows these folks coming in the door for treatment don't have much of anything and certainly don't have the money to pay deductibles and out-of-pocket expenses. There are companies who choose to write this off, and there are companies who choose to act like every dollar is gold. I was not going to tolerate that, so I started sneaking my clients in the side door after group started so they did not have to walk by Human Resources.

Eventually, the SUD supervisor moved me to the downtown location, so people wouldn't have to tolerate me out there, and I wouldn't have to tolerate them. They also had no caffeine on campus and clients did not like that. So, I took my clients, and we moved back to town—the migration continued. This location was so much better and much more laid back. People interacted with each other, and there was a homeless team working at this location. They were a humble lot. This place was a vibrant location, with a lot of moving parts. They welcomed me and gave me what I needed, as they understood this gave their program some extra clients for therapy and ARHMS workers and case management. The folks at the downtown location felt the same way about the campus in general, so we got along great.

Now, as you read this, you are probably thinking that this writer is like a bull in a china shop and creates chaos wherever he goes. That is a fair assessment, if you don't know me. I can be difficult to work with, but there is a reason for that. I have been around the block enough as an addict and professional to know what is right, and I am going to voice my opinions, especially when there are people being deceptive, people not operating with integrity, and people taking advantage of clients. I go to bat for my clients and fight for them. I fight for their rights when no one else does. And I know most of them have nothing, so I am not going to take their money when they have mouths to feed. That is what insurance is for. When I worked for a satellite office in St. Peter, I heard a story about the man who previously owned the place and had his office at the "mothership" in Waverly. He had twenty-four male residential beds, but he also had "the twenty-fifth bed." This bed was always filled, but it was a bed that was never billed. This bed was for clients who had no insurance and couldn't pay $30,000 for an inpatient stay. He filled this bed with thirteen and a half clients each year and ate the cost. Counselors had to do the paperwork, of course, but the client was given free treatment. This is called integrity, and I told myself at the time that if I had the opportunity to once again run a treatment program, I was going to scholarship clients as well. I am not about the money, and I have proven that to the population I serve over and over again. In my role as Clinical Supervisor and Treatment Director, I had the pleasure of shredding deductible invoices in front of the client, so they wouldn't have to pay. It made me feel so good (the client as well). I am not hard to work with when I find someone who puts the client first and their ego second. Plus, I made facilities a lot of money, as my groups were monstrous, and I was willing to work weekends to get all the paperwork done.

When I moved to the downtown location, I felt like I could breathe. The campus was stifling me, and there was a "hovering" there that just made me feel like no one trusted anyone. The HR people were money hungry and would take a client's last dollar. There were too many people that worked there that did not do any billable services, and they needed to get paid. Have you ever worked for a place where ten percent of the people made all the money for the company, and the other ninety percent sat around all day in meetings and accomplished nothing? That was the feeling I got out there. At the downtown location, it felt real. Everybody worked, and the place had a "fun" feel. I enjoyed it. More importantly, the clients enjoyed it. They thought it was so much better than the plastic environment the campus provided. The year turned over to 2019, and the methodical five-year master's grind came to a close.

My Master's Degree and a New/Old Opportunity

I finished my internship at Blue Stem after nine months and received my master's degree on my fifty-first birthday —February 10th, 2019. It was a very proud moment for me, without a lot of fanfare. I thought about showing up and walking at graduation, but it was in Washington DC, and I didn't want to spend another nickel on college. The degree cost me $60,000. That wasn't the end of it, though. If you want to have the mental health license that goes with the degree, you have to do two years of clinical supervision with a "board licensed" clinician. I could have done this for free at my current work site. However, I had made some good connections at my internship site and chose to pay to work with someone I knew could teach me a lot about mental health and the therapy aspect of counseling. I started that in April of 2019 and paid out of pocket for the two years of supervision (roughly $7,000). I have to say that this is where integrity plays a big role in my recovery. I know specific cases of people doing supervision at their places of employment, and they get to "slide by" by not completing their allotted hours, not having to do the full two years, etc. By doing this the right way, it gave me a profound sense of gratitude for my recovery program, as my days of cheating the system were over. I knew that the two years were going to be long, but patience is a virtue, and I know that today. I learned a lot about personality disorders through the two years, as "Dr. B" worked with borderline personality disorders as her specialty, and this helped my practice. Doing life "the right way" instead of the easy way has been the story of my recovery. There isn't much that has ever been handed to me, and for that, I am grateful.

On January 1st, 2019, the first New Year's message I received was from my old "boss," whose business was struggling. My replacement lasted about three and a half months, and she decided that the job wasn't what she wanted. They were desperate to get me back. The financial aspect of the company was crumbling, and they were bringing in about twenty-five percent of what I did. The text was half-apology for the way she treated me and half, "are you interested in coming back?" I went out for lunch with her in March, and we talked about business, and she asked me if I wanted to come back. She had purchased more of the building and was in the process of moving the treatment to one side of the building, eliminating chaos and disorder. She also hired people to construct a group room the way I dreamed of, with couches, soft chairs, and an aura of welcoming, rather than the institution feel that makes up treatment group rooms in a lot of places. I mulled her offer, and we met three more times before I made the decision to come back. It was a relief putting in my notice, and I told myself this would be my last addictions related job in Rochester. I lugged all my clients back to where they came from and started back on July 1st, 2019. We had made the entire loop around Rochester! My employer did not try to keep me and allowed me to go with no argument. I think he was tired of trying to appease the Human Resources department, as they complained about me to him on many occasions. I actually would call in the supervisor to listen to my conversations with HR on speaker, so she knew I was acting respectfully. This opened their eyes and ears to the truth, as HR would later say I was rude during our conversations, and I had eyewitnesses who heard the entirety of the phone call exchange. It was so unbearable that it just had to end. There were so many meetings to attend, and many made no sense. If you asked what the reasoning was for this meeting or this workshop, they would come up with some statement like, "this is the way we have always done it." I left there on June 28th and came back to the treatment program I started and was met with open arms.

The Second Stint – Eighth Counseling Job

I brought all of my clients back here from my previous employer, and that place faded from my memory fast. I had now taken many of my clients on a tour of Rochester, and some of them had moved locations with me all four times. I had not been asked to sign a "no compete," which would have prohibited this. I had to re-admit all of the clients, which took time, but soon I was up and running, with a new group room, new set of offices, and new salary. I walked away from drug court with a change in employment, and this was the best thing I could have done. I had stopped enjoying drug court long before that, as it was just so different than the other drug courts I had worked for. There was just too much drama, and I did not feel like my voice was being heard, like I did in the other two. There were too many papers to write for sanctions, and not enough swift, short jail sanctions, in my opinions. I had one client who told me that he used alcohol throughout the entirety of his drug court stint because he was in there for methamphetamines, and they would give him a "quick test" and then throw it away. I lasted there 27 months. As for my new gig, the clients appreciated the fresh start, including the large, open group room, which was conducive to recovery. I had found out that while I was gone, the person who had briefly taken my place had tried to completely change the program, including the online documents for paperwork. She wanted to put her stamp on it, I guess. However, it made for a lot of confusion, and it created more paperwork. It took time to set things right. I was given autonomy, and people stayed out of my way for the first year, letting me do what I do. I was good at it because I worked at it—hard. I worked almost every Saturday for almost ten years straight, as I had large groups and a lot of paperwork. This takes a massive amount of discipline, and if there are counselors reading this book, they are nodding their heads right now. What is often ignored in addiction counseling college programs is the massive amount of paperwork that is required of licensed counselors. There cannot be interruptions, people walking in unannounced to see you, or other disturbances. I asked for locks to be installed to keep clients at bay, as in the past, they could just walk right back to my office and knock on the door. This new system created more of a professional environment. There was a chance to have some barriers in place, so clients had to check in up front and not just come and interrupt counselors at work. This is the way to protect counselors and allow them to get tasks done. Things changed—for a while. The first year went very well, and things returned to normal at my "new, old job." I was bringing the program back to life, the place filled up, and the entire setup felt different. There was less noise, and my office was set up way in the back of the new side, which gave me (and my clients) some privacy. I was back running full groups immediately and even started a Step-Down group and my first alumni group by the end of 2019. By now, I had established a reputation through my years in counseling, as former clients that got clean would recommend me and talk about me to their friends and addicts that were struggling. The word had spread in the community and we became prosperous. This was the first time I had really noticed this since I had come back to Rochester three years ago. Life became extremely busy as I was in the midst of my clinical supervision for my LPCC, working sixty hours per week and lacking in self-care. My balance just plain sucked, so, 2019 became the year that I decided to redo the steps of AA with a new sponsor.

I began to work with a sponsor in the fall of 2018, and when he left to go south for the winter, I was punted off to one of his "sponsees," a retired social worker at Mayo. I had gone through steps one through four with "Bob" and completed my fifth step with "Mike" on January 5th, 2019. He asked me after this if I had ever heard of the book, *Drop the Rock*. As fate would have it, someone had given me the book years ago when she graduated from the Hazelden program and donated many other books. I had it right on the shelf, although I had never even picked it up. This book is a ninety-three-page life changer about working the sixth and seventh steps, which are somewhat glossed over in the *Big Book*. We started to dissect the book in January of 2019, and we finished in August of 2020. This book had the same effect on me that the first 164 pages of the *Big Book* did back in 2007-08. It was a book that described these steps as action steps, and they deal with character defects that "maximize" during years of drinking but can crop up (or remain) in sobriety and turn people into "dry drunks." This book was a lifesaver to me and helped me get into a better balance and frame of mind. It helped me reframe a lot of my skewed perspectives and perceptions. Going through this book methodically helped me digest a few pages or paragraphs each week and apply them to my life. It led the way for me to reinvest in going to church, which is now part of my Sunday "trifecta," which includes AA, church, and the gym. It also led me to read the sequel to *Drop the Rock,* which is called *The Ripple Effect.* This sequel is about using step ten to work steps six and seven every day. I mention this because it is this work with a sponsor and continued work with the steps that has allowed this alcoholic and drug addict to not only survive but thrive in the professional world of addictions counseling. As life caromed toward the absolute devastation of 2020, my life was getting to be in a good place. My career outline was taking shape. I was set to teach my first class at Winona State University in 2020, I was set up to take the Mental Health Clinical test, I was thriving in my job, my balance was getting slowly better, and I was starting to put my life in order after twelve years of sobriety. My job was rewarding in its autonomy, and running my own program and curriculum was very satisfying. The outcomes were good, and I started believing in myself more. I had transformed my life and was even becoming joyous at times. I even put aside my long resentment against my former employer, setting up a meeting with him and shaking his hand. Most importantly, I finally started believing that I was a good man. This had hampered me for years because of past mistakes and numerous marches before judges. As 2020 began, no one could see the craziness that was about to engulf us, and it set the tone for a very interesting year.

March 20th, 2020

I went and saw the death metal band Vader on February 21st, 2020, and there were no indications at that time of what was to come. People were smashed into The Varsity Theater like sardines to see these stalwarts, and there was no talk at all about COVID-19. When March rolled around, it became the talk of the world, and soon after my family group in March, which was attended by over fifty people, the state of Minnesota went into lockdown. Businesses were forced to close, and only "essential" workers were allowed to keep their lights on. This created a huge conundrum for treatment providers. What do you do? Are we essential, or do we need to go to Telehealth computer services to connect with our clients? The decisions were ultimately made by each individual agency and treatment provider, and this next section of the book is something I am quite proud of.

As people headed to the grocery stores to rip all the toilet paper off the shelves, hunker down at home, and wait for the next directive by the government, I made the decision to stay open for face-to-face treatment groups. I can't speak for every treatment program in the state, but I can tell you that every other organization I knew went to Telehealth—aka Zoom meetings. My experience in attending AA meetings and my reliance on face-to-face groups led the way. However, just as important to me was the fact that I was no longer going to live life in fear, like I had done for so long when I was drinking, smoking crack, and breaking the law. My choice was easy, so action was taken on the fly. We cleaned the hell out of that group room twice per day, and I divided my group into two groups to lessen the size, and I stayed open. This was once again deemed controversial by some agencies, as "Tim was putting people at risk." Listen, if you have learned one thing from reading this book, it is that I don't really care what people think of me, as I operate from my value system, which is embedded in recovery principles. My long-term clients told me they would rather get COVID than relapse back into active addiction, and I was not going to abandon them during this pandemic. Addiction and mental health disorders breed in isolation, and this is exactly what the government was telling people to do—don't leave your house, and we will pay you to do it. It was a recipe for disaster. . .So, I stayed open. People who had any symptoms were told to stay home, and many got tested. However, there were no positive cases that stemmed from the treatment center, and we just kept at it. The medicine for addiction is face-to-face meetings and the group milieu. This is what it is all about. Staying open was the only option for me, and pretty soon, two local television stations took some interest in my group and how things were going, as they were desperate for positive stories during this nightmare. One television station did an interview in July and followed up with "The Twelve Days of Christmas," where they interviewed twelve of my clients who had between nine months and two years of sobriety. They all stated that face-to-face meetings and being connected during this pandemic were the most important parts of staying sober in 2020. Now, of course, this created more controversy, but by this time, I was actually becoming immune to it. It was all just "white noise." The clients were appreciative, and something very amazing was slowly taking place, day by day and week by week. This group of humans were bonding and connecting during a pandemic, and they were staying sober. Not just one or two of them, but over twenty clients (twenty-four, to be exact) began a sustained life of recovery during this time. The proof was in the pudding, so to speak. Connection is the antidote to addiction. In a world where people were getting paid to stay home and being told to stay away from other humans, this group of people were connecting nine to ten hours per week, staying sober, and getting their families back in the fold. It was a huge win for the "pandemic twenty," the moniker I used for this group that has sustained their sobriety. More on this later.

COVID and 2020 –
The Year of Two Pandemics

COVID-19 has ravaged the world, no doubt, but there was another pandemic going on in 2020, and that was unchecked drug and alcohol abuse. Inpatient treatment centers were running with some limitations, but outpatient addiction treatment and mental health services had gone the route of Telehealth. This is an ineffective way to do treatment, as face-to-face meetings are where the real magic happens. It is better than nothing, but barely. In the city of Rochester, the pandemic had led to the utilization of Telehealth services for most programs, and some took over one year to return to face-to-face meetings. When providers sent their people home to do treatment in front of a computer screen, many clients relapsed within hours. I know because I admitted some to my group. This put me in a precarious situation, as there are many providers who have lost huge sums of money due to empty treatment rooms, the weakness of Telehealth services, and the lack of community accountability. This created a lot of stress and a lot of jealousy and anger in the community. People were fatigued with wearing masks, social distancing, and staying apart from others, and this led to a lot of overt hostility. As I write this section at the end of November of 2020, the year has been one huge mess. Concerts I had paid for and were readying for had been canceled or postponed, there have been lockdowns, gyms and AA clubs have been closed for months, and people are drinking, using drugs and selling drugs, unchecked. My decision to stay open and provide face-to-face treatment services has been deemed controversial by some "professionals." It has been an easy sell for my clients, as many of them have flourished during this time of taking away liberties and rights that American citizens deserve. In the community, on the other hand, it has been a source of contention for some providers and probation officers. This plague has given many active addicts a chance to crawl back into the shell of learned helplessness, which included taking advantage of the system. By giving clients a place to go to during this time, it allowed them an identity, and a purpose, which is to be a part of a group. People stayed clean, and took weekly, witnessed urine screens to back this up. This gives me a great sense of joy and has made the decision to stay open and put myself at risk an easy one. I have been called a risk taker, selfish, and many other names by people in the profession, but none of this mattered when my passion is strong for helping others. I worked with forty clients in two groups, including many who met with me individually. I created an alumni group that meets weekly, and staying open gave accountability to clients. I have run three family groups and continue to be one of the few programs to run live groups since the start of COVID—perhaps in the state (this section was written at the end of 2020). This has been confirmed by many inpatient treatment counselors who are looking for aftercare for their clients. They state they know of no other outpatient program that was running face-to-face meetings unless they have groups of three to six. What exacerbates the situation is that probation pretty much ceased operations in 2020, as POs worked from home, which meant that there were no urine tests, and their clients had a free pass. I became the counselor, PO, Child Protection Worker, and main source of client accountability. There were phone calls to the facility weekly, where people would complain that clients were not wearing masks, they were not social distancing, and there were too many people in the group, blah, blah, blah. It has really hardened me as a person to have to live through all the discontent and bitterness of some people in this profession. The goal for me has simply always been this: I want to help as many clients as I can and provide the ethical, quality, evidence-based-treatment, to give them the best chance to succeed. I will not let it take my joy, but it has stopped me from collaborating with agencies face-to-face and has stopped me from going to several provider meetings in the community. I just cannot walk into a place where there have been complaints made against me time and time again and then have them come up and attempt to shake my hand with a smile on their face. It is disheartening to see people act this way. They know who they are. At the end of the Covid run, I felt like my decision was sound and strong, and the end result was that many people stayed sober. This is all that matters.

The Rest of 2020

This year was also a year of accomplishment, as I passed the National Clinical Mental Health Counseling Exam on October 6th. I studied laboriously for six months prior to taking it because I heard the horror stories about the difficulties of this exam and how many times some people had to take it. I was going to be "one and done," and that is what happened, as I passed it with a lot of room to spare. However, I made daily deposits towards this for six months, which allowed me to take out the withdrawal. That was a huge step for me, and it showed me once again that I belong in the mental health field of professionals. When the year ended, I had brought in almost $300,000 for the organization, and this was despite the scholarships that I provided. Yes, I gave people that were struggling financially free treatment! I had a strong year employment-wise, and handled the year with some courage. At the end of the year, a local TV station wanted to end 2020 on a positive note, and they took the time to go in-depth with fifteen of my clients who stayed sober during 2020 and were about to spend the holidays with their families. It was a well-done piece.

"The Pandemic Twenty" from 2020-2021

I wanted to go back to the face-to-face meetings in 2020 for a minute because it reinforces a valuable lesson I learned a long time ago. What keeps people sober? There are a lot of answers to that question, but the simple answer for me is connection. I read the Rat Park experiment about social connection and Johann Hari's article about connection, and I jumped on that train right away because I lived it and saw the power of connection in early recovery. When the pandemic hit and our governor shut down the state except for "essential services," I knew this was going to be a horror show for many people in recovery. I saw almost all AA meetings go to Zoom, and outpatient treatment became "Telehealth." It was fear, and people bought into that fear factor one hundred percent. I am sure other treatment professionals made the connection between isolation and addiction, but facility directors ordered them to begin Telehealth sessions. Our famous hospital was included among the culprits that sent their patients home with no follow-up care. I ended up with three of them who were lucky enough to get in after relapses. I was not going to abandon my clients and spend the year looking at them through a computer screen. That is such a weak way to do treatment. I told them that I was going to stay open for face-to-face meetings, and we were going to divide the group into two groups because of the recommendations of only having ten in a room indoors. I doubled my group hours to make this feasible. When I looked back at my client list in 2020, I had between forty-one and forty-five clients in programming with me and running two separate groups on multiple days. My clients appreciated this immensely. We reframed from "I have to go to treatment" to "I GET to go to treatment." People bought in and rallied around each other. They found places that were open for face-to-face meetings (Celebrate Recovery, AA, NA, etc.) and caravanned to these places. They held each other accountable. They were two to three urine screens each week. We did family groups for the people willing to leave the house. My treatment clients watched addiction take hold of the community and do serious damage just as it did elsewhere. However, they had the group, the support, and each other. I have never had another group like this, and now I know I never will again due to the circumstances. I have had twenty-four people out of this group of clients make it through the years of 2020-2021, not just sober but in recovery. Most of them are still sober today (it is now June of 2022), and I know this because they continue to come in, speak to my current groups, go to alumni groups, attend my mental wellness groups, and stay connected. The number "twenty-four" paints a solid picture of how important it is to have that connection and how this group battled together in a pandemic year to stay sober and get their lives back. These folks have created a positive ripple effect in the community with their families, employers, and addicts looking for a way out. Many of them sponsor today, and others became Peer Recovery Coaches or went back to school to become helping professionals. When I take the time to think about this, I realize how important it was for people to get together and connect, and that a simple group room could become that place. Clients who had been to twenty inpatient treatments were able to sustain their sobriety in a world where many things were just ripped from humans, like the gym, meetings, social events, etc. This is definitely the highlight of my counseling career, and when I look back at this, I know it will never be duplicated (at least by me). As I write this section, it is the end of 2021, I just had a holiday party for this group, and fifty people showed up. A picture is included in this book as I wanted to really emphasize that this group did amazing work, and they did it during a pandemic and in the community. I just graduated out the last of them, although many of them will continue on in some fashion with me. I want to take the time right here to thank every one of them. This was the biggest joy in my counseling career.

My Work Ethic

If someone enters the field of addiction counseling and works their way up the ladder, they already know it takes a lot of hours to complete the work if they want to be effective and help many people. This is where my self-discipline comes into play. I have worked most holidays and holiday weekends, including Memorial Day, July 4th, Thanksgiving, Christmas Eve, New Year's Eve, and Labor Day. Holidays are paperwork days for me, and people who work in this field will understand that. I am known for having large group sizes, but there is a price to pay for facilitating large groups. The paperwork portion of this job is immense. I have averaged over fifty hours per week for the last twelve years and have taken three vacations. I have sacrificed a lot in the name of helping others, and my self-care has been poor in the past. I am working on this now, but my work ethic has been a huge factor in my ability to learn and grow in this field.

I must also mention group size here, and this is another controversial subject that has followed me around the city where I work. The DHS has rules and statutes we must follow, and one of them is that there cannot be more than sixteen clients in a group at any given time. DHS wants counselors to have a caseload of no more than that. Anyone who has worked in this field for any amount of time understands that getting seventy percent of clients to show up consistently is a great rate. This would be an average of eleven clients per day, which is a nice-sized group for most people, but I have never been content with helping such a small amount of people. I average about eighteen to twenty clients per day and have ever since I started counseling in 2012. This is often scoffed at by professionals, stating that there are too many in the group. My PG-13 answer to that is that I keep them for twelve to eighteen months, and it is virtually impossible to slip between the cracks during that time. Clients are tested for substances two to three times per week. I also do not bill for more than sixteen in a group, so every once in a while, someone gets a free day of treatment services. This is not about the money—this is about helping others to the best of my ability. Now, this creates a lot of animosity amongst money whores in the field, but there are some people who can thrive in this environment and make this work. However, as I sit here writing this book, I have to tell you that it has taken its toll. I have sacrificed a lot in the name of paperwork and helping others, and all those years of massive amounts of paperwork have taken their toll. My work ethic is strong, but I think I have proved to others that I am not lazy. I am just slowing down. My cup is getting empty earlier and earlier in the week. There are many reasons why people do not do long-term outpatient treatment, and the biggest reason is that you get invested in the clients, and many of them break your heart. It is a difficult task, and it has the ability to wear someone down to a nub.

2021—
Death Comes to my Front Door

This year has been a tough one for me, as I lost both my mother and my father in the first four months of the year. My mother passed on February 6th, and my father on April 3rd of 2021. I was there at the end for both of them, and my recovery program helped me to be able to absorb these losses. However, no one else from my family stepped in and helped, which made this very difficult. Losing them both in a short period of time was harder on me than I thought, but it was a gift to be able to be there at the end for both my mother and father. I have both of their urns at home, so they are always with me. Recovery has allowed me to forgive my mother, and surprisingly, I wept like a baby at the end, sitting in the Domitillo Building at Mayo and watching her last breaths. To add to the misery of the beginning of this year, a client of mine for three years overdosed and died on May 27th, 2021, after twenty-one months of sustained sobriety. He used heroin once, and that was all it took. This has made this year a heavy year for me and it took away some of the ecstasy from finally be awarded my Licensed Professional Clinical Counselor (LPCC) license on June 11th, 2021. It is still fresh in my mind, getting that in the mail and how much effort went into earning that piece of paper. My LADC license is #303329, and my LPCC license is #2873. That is quite the difference!!! The work that went into this license was a lot, and a lot of sacrifices have been made over the past seven years. This is going to open doors for me that I never thought possible, such as working in private practice without all the red tape. It is exciting to get the reward after trudging through the past seven years, not really seeing the finish line, or looking at the possibilities with a dual license. It is so nice to have options and not to be stuck because at some point, I knew I was going to walk away from the field of addictions. It is too heartbreaking, and there is a serious lack of reward. There is a heaviness to working in this field that goes beyond compassion fatigue into emotional numbness and exhaustion. I am talking about community recovery, not working for some conglomerate where you are shielded from everything. I am talking about "here-and-now" crisis situations that come in off the street for help. It tires people out, especially someone who is in recovery from alcohol and drugs. It has been over a twelve-year run!!! I love working with people trying to find recovery, but the paperwork demands are outrageous. I also work with a lot of interns, and they tire me out as well. That's another reason why the shelf life for an addictions counselor is about three years. It is a tiring, low-paying job, and compassion fatigue is a very real dilemma. Most people I have talked to that have worked in the addictions field stated they waited about one to two years too long before branching out into something else or, at least, changing environments. I am feeling that amidst the Covid pandemic, the endless fifty-hour weeks, the multiple responsibilities, and the multiple agencies I have toiled for, it has all caught up to me. I still have high energy and I still have the passion, but at the end of the week, I am shot. There is a saying that you cannot pour from an empty cup, which means that you have to have your cup filled to be able to help others. Mine was empty by the middle of the week at times, and I had to tap that reservoir that allows one to go on autopilot. My time in this field was entering the final act.

2021 –
The Second Half of the Year—I'm Done, Man

The first half of 2021 was a culmination of sadness, accomplishment, and heartache. The second half of the year was tough as well, but for different reasons. Some changes were happening at work, including the resignation of the CEO, who was also the founder of the company. I made my pitch for a raise after I received my LPCC, as my intention was to start the mental health component at this facility. I was not being greedy but rather, looking at the sacrifices of the past seven years. I had worked almost every Saturday, holiday, and other days that end in "Y" for the past two years. I had brought in about $825,000 in four years, and this gave the facility flexibility. This small company needs employees to earn, or it goes down in flames, simple as that. Now that I had a mental health license, there was an opportunity to become a dual-diagnosis facility, where we could work with both the addiction piece and the mental health. Most, if not all, of the other agencies in town were dual diagnosis centers, and this was a way to keep everything in-house, and become a more legitimate company. It would also give the agency more financial flexibility, as we could bill an enhanced rate for the dual diagnosis license. However, the ball was dropped on sending the co-occurring enhancement rate to the DHS, and this delayed the opportunity for the organization to make money. The Board of Directors, who I had not even met but once over four years, decided to have five of my co-workers fill out a performance evaluation on me prior to being considered for a raise. One of the co-workers crucified me and stated I was a poor leader and did not validate them enough. This co-worker did her 880- hour internship with me, has an office right next to me and was given an amazing evaluation by "yours truly" after her internship was completed. I hired her, had recently given her a raise, and heaped praise on her, often. To say I was shocked was an understatement. When I read the overall summation of the performance review, that piece of it made me physically sick. I was a sixty-hour-work-week guy, week after week, kept four group rooms full, and this company was financially fit. This raise was about more than the money. It was about respect, and I felt like my inventory was taken by anonymous people in the most cowardly way possible. The person who made these comments anonymously (I found out who it was—it was not hard) had many opportunities to come into my office and talk to me about her viewpoints. She did 880 internship hours with me, and that takes time and sacrifice. However, this is just the nature of the business. It is cut-throat, and it is unhealthy as hell. I would never do this to anyone else, and there is a certain recurring theme in this manuscript that continues to rear its ugly head. People like to stab in the back, and once again, there was targeting at play. I have an open-door policy, and this person could have come in and talked to me about their contentions, and I would have listened, and we could have worked it out. However, to do this in a review knowing the damage it was going to do, was unacceptable and unprofessional. Knowing there was someone in the company that tossed that grenade made it impossible to come to work every day without some level of frustration. Have you ever pulled up to your place of employment and saw the car of a co-worker, which elicited a cringe? That was me. To add another layer of absurdity on top of this, there is a certain board member who was brought in by the former CEO (best friends—another atrocity), that was absolutely against me getting a raise. She is a person that identifies herself as "in recovery" but harbors resentments against me. She knows how many people I have helped, but what she does not know is how much time I put into my education and advancing my career, to be able to better help clients in need. She did not want me to have a raise, so she voiced that. So… add up all the layers and layers of sickness and drama and ego and chaos and competition, and…that was it. I made up my mind that my days working in an addiction treatment setting in Rochester were done. I had had it. That was the last straw. I put in my resignation in the middle of November, with my last day being December 31st, 2021. It was time to move on to the next chapter (therapy, adjunct teaching, supervision, and speaking engagements). The last twelve years of working in various treatment centers has hardened me as a human, and it has nothing to do with the clients. They are actually what kept me in the field for as long as I was. This is about some of the people who worked alongside me. I have never seen anything like it. When I was teaching, there was a modicum of professionalism no matter where I subbed or taught. I had probably been to thirty different schools, and they were all good people. Maybe I got spoiled and had expectations. I think it just dawned on me as I have been writing this over the past six years that every day has taken a little bit of me, and all the little jabs have taken their toll. I have just had enough. It is time to drop the big rock I have been carrying around that has caused much anguish for me and for the people I call my friends and family. There is no award for counselor of the year, and I have spent many years working toward this mystical award, pushing myself harder and harder until there is really nothing left of me. I am sure, one day, I will thank the person who hammered me on my performance evaluation (as well as the board member), because that is what it has taken for me to finally wake up and realize this life is just too damn short and I want to be happier. God has a funny way of hinting at me to make changes and then finally just using blunt force trauma to get His point through my thick skull. I needed to get out of this field before it ruins me. Message received!!!!

PART III

State of the Treatment Profession: Some Good, Some Bad, and Some Solutions

As you have read up to this point (it is now 2022), I have worked in all milieus, including residential, outpatient, and sober housing. I have now worked at eight different agencies (two agencies I worked at twice), and have worked continuously as a LADC since 2010 (including one year of internship). I have worked with adolescents and adults, men and women. I have worked with three county drug courts and have run both traditional outpatient and long-term outpatient programs. I have started four programs since I was licensed, including an opioid-specific program, an adolescent outpatient program, and two long-term intensive outpatient treatment programs. I have finished a master's degree in Addiction Counseling, am a Licensed Professional Clinical Counselor, A Licensed Alcohol and Drug Counselor, and I have my Clinical Supervision certificate. Most importantly, I have facilitated over 2,000 groups and admitted over 1200 clients in the past twelve years. I believe I am more than equipped to give my opinion on the treatment milieu from my little corner of the world, and even though this might not be true in other areas, this is what I have seen from my experience. I think it is of great importance to know the truth about treatment from an insider's perspective, similar to what Anne Fletcher did in her book, *Inside Rehab*. My years in the trenches have given me many startling revelations, and so I am going to speak on the state of the profession and to offer some potential solutions. They are my opinions only, but I think they have value, and in the right hands, can be helpful when starting an organization working with people suffering from substance use disorders.

Long-Term Intensive Outpatient Treatment is Gold With the Right "Teacher"

I was working in St. Peter with drug court participants in 2014-2015 and became fascinated with long-term outpatient treatment. In my first counseling job, I had the tendency to keep patients for a long time, up to nine months, especially those who were not willing to go to AA. I hadn't really thought much about it, as it seemed normal to me, but now I see the writing on the wall. Some of these participants were in treatment for one year, and although they were only coming once per week, I saw the results. I started to research retention in treatment and saw there was a direct correlation between time spent in treatment and sustained sobriety. However, the hard part is to keep them engaged long-term, as I have found that many "tap out." My opioid group died two months after I left, and another facility even tried to take this on after I left. They called, and I gave them my curriculum for a cup of coffee at Dunn Brothers. They failed because they had the wrong person facilitating. People are not going to buy into long-term programming when the facilitator is dry and not reaching the clients. I started looking around the state for long-term intensive outpatient treatment (IOP), and I found one in Rochester, but that one was a corrections-based treatment, and I wanted one that was mostly probation free. I developed one in St. Peter in 2016 and it flourished. I later moved to Rochester and began a long-term IOP in 2017 and ran it through 2021. The other long-term IOP in Rochester folded in 2018, so my program became relatively unique. Now, I am not going to sugarcoat this. It is extremely hard to run and very frustrating at times. The reason is that there is no real "blueprint" that I know of to follow, which means that facilitators have to collaborate, get supervision, and bounce ideas off other professionals incessantly. The bottom line is that the reasons to run a long-term IOP are plentiful, although it takes someone with a lot of passion and is person-centered. Here are some of the reasons. Long-term outpatient treatment is perfect for "revolving door" clients who have recycled in and out of treatment most of their lives. These folks need a lot of time for healing, whether we are talking about the brain, spiritual healing, emotional healing, etc. We have to look at the clients who are going to twenty-plus treatments and stop this nonsense. Long-term community-based IOP is a solution for those willing to "peel back and unpack" the layers of trauma, loss, self-esteem erosion, and emotional dysregulation that is often required to make someone whole again. These traditional outpatient treatment programs run between three and four months, and many times clients are given a number of hours to complete. Once they complete them, treatment is done. I have never understood that, and I can't even begin to fathom what programs are thinking when they graduate people out of outpatient at around three or four months of sobriety. This is the time when clients are starting to feel emotions, and because they have been numbing their feelings for so long, they often take up the bottle again or the drugs.

Researchers state that post-acute-withdrawal syndrome (PAWS) often reaches its peak at six months of sobriety. This is the time to add services to the mix, such as therapy, as well as sponsorship. Long-term IOP can be a "tiered" approach and tapered over the twelve to eighteen months as people start to grow in their recovery. PAWS is very real, and it can take from eighteen to twenty-four months for the brain to heal, so I keep them as long as I can and then shoot them into an alumni group. This gives the client a fighting chance. Remember, when many of these folks come into treatment, they have lost their jobs, their homes, their kids, their driver's licenses, their dignity, and self-worth. They are at a very low place, and three months isn't going to fix that. Three months is going to put a band-aid on all the problems, which will be summarily ripped off as soon as they lose the accountability of the program. Now, many clients will "tap out" or walk away from the program before they are done. That is because of patterns in their past where they do well for a period of time and then just get overwhelmed with handling all aspects of their life sober. They are used to responding to success with sabotage. They are welcomed back, and many will reach back out after another disastrous run. I also coin people out early, sometimes at eight to ten months, because they have reached their therapeutic peak. However, most of the clients I admit are fifteen to twenty-lifetime treatment folks, and they need the accountability of long-term programming— in the community. They need the structure, and they need to learn the grit and self-discipline to stay the course. Recovery is based on routine and creating new neurological pathways in the brain. This is done by walking a new path through the creation of new routines and habits. It takes time, and patience is a virtue.

The importance of urine screens cannot be overstated, and two witnessed urine tests per week for the first six months are highly recommended. Some clients take three. This adds another layer of accountability, as clients know that Mondays are testing days, and it gives them some added weekend protection. Many clients WANT to be held accountable—remember that. At one facility I worked at, the CEO stated they won't do urine tests because they don't want the clients to leave the program. This is a telling sign that treatment is disguised as a money-making venture. The CEO does not want her clients to get better, nor does she understand the first thing about treatment accountability. Her client base is ninety percent probation clients as well, and they need the accountability.

The topics, or cognitive-behavioral therapy-based learning modules, as I call them, are practical, and there are some "usual suspects" here, such as healthy boundaries, cognitive distortions (thinking errors), reframing, codependency, handling cravings, impulse control, etc. However, I also incorporate some other areas of recovery that many SUD clients know nothing about. Some of these include a unit on nutrition, physical health, financial planning, mental toughness, self-discipline, grit, environmental wellness, healthy relationships, etc. There is a heavy element of family sessions, family education, and family therapy. There is a dual-licensed group facilitator, as almost all these clients have co-occurring disorders. We talk about the importance of connection and how vital it is in recovery. If someone is willing, they can be provided with a recovery coach, a sponsor, a therapist, a counselor, and a supportive group of peers in the later stages of treatment or an alumni group. These serve as guides for all the different life problems, and the more of these valuable people, the better. This takes an army, or "recovery herd." It's all about staying connected.

Master's Degrees are Vital

When I began working with clients who suffer from substance use disorders, I came at this with a lot of passion and motivation, which helped me form therapeutic relationships. My years of teaching experience helped me with the education part of addictions treatment, and I had no fear as a group facilitator. I obtained a twenty-four-credit "Graduate Certificate" that qualified me to be a LADC, which included an 880-hour internship. Needless to say, I didn't know what the hell I was doing, but I sure thought I did. In the world of addiction counseling in the state of Minnesota, the amount of education needed is startling. For example, a young adult student can take the LADC core classes (six in all), do an internship, get an associate's degree, and become an addictions counselor with the designation called "Alcohol and Drug Counselor—Temporary License," or ADC-T. It is not uncommon to see young counselors coming into the field of counseling with minimal life experience, no experience working with clients with substance use disorders, and coming off an internship where interns are actually doing the job of the counselor, who in turn, is scrambling to get paperwork done. There is little learning involved, and most counselors do not want the "baggage" of an intern. The reason for this is simple: Counselors have so much paperwork to do, and interns fall through the cracks. I have supervised twenty-two interns and have a lot of experience working with them. However, they are a lot of work if you invest in them. If you don't, they go out into the counseling world like lambs to the slaughter. I vividly remember my first day of interning in 2010—I walked in the door, and within five minutes, I was on my own. I was interning at a residential treatment center attached to a hospital, so there were a lot of employees. No one even told me where to put my coat or my backpack. I ended up following the clients around all day, and several staff members later told me they thought I was a new client they hadn't met yet. I was later told by my supervisor that this was a test because of the large volume of interns they have in their company. It was a "weeding out" process, and he told me that some interns in the past have just walked out and went home, frustrated and in tears. That was the first of many "head scratchers" for me. Companies often take advantage of interns and bill for everything they do. When I was finishing my 880-hour internship at a different place, I was running my supervisor's treatment group while she sat in the office trying to get caught up on paperwork. This went on and on for two months. Looking back on this, I am just grateful that I was forty years old and I had some life experiences, and some common sense. I never questioned anything, but I certainly remember saying to myself, "This is so messed up."

Once the internship is completed, you are often hired on for a minimal wage, and as in any profession, you get what you pay for. They stick a young person with a two-year degree in a room with criminal addicts (as many as they can pile in there). Counselors end up doing unintentional harm, getting manipulated and don't even realize it. It is a broken system. Clients do not get what they need. Some ADC-T's do not know how to form simple sentences, as their grammar is lacking, and their writing looks a lot like a text message. I have seen run-on paragraphs without any periods. This is a bad look when paperwork is seventy percent of the job (which many counselors-in-training are blindsided by because they were not informed of the heavy weight put on paperwork in this profession). Some of these "counselors" walk away from the field due to the paperwork, but many soldier on, causing harm such as boundary violations. A master's degree should be required to work with difficult clients with co-occurring disorders, and a dual license should be preferred. Anything less is dangerous. I would not have believed the importance of this early on in my counseling career, but the need for a master's degree is obvious for a number of reasons. A master's degree will force professionals to become better writers, and this is paramount. I do not want a document from a facility I work at to go to another professional with a multitude of mistakes, poor sentence construction, and that lacks professionalism in all aspects. It is a bad look for everyone involved. A second reason is the sheer enormity of clients who walk in the door with co-occurring mental health disorders. A master's program will give students plenty of education on dual diagnoses, and that is vital in treating the entire person. A master's degree will also teach students discipline, which is important in getting paperwork done. This is a big problem in the world of addiction counseling. A master's degree will also give students a chance to do multiple internships, which adds perspective and different approaches. The supervision aspect of a master's internship (and subsequence clinical supervision) is a great learning experience. Finally, students (especially those in recovery) will learn more about professionalism, working as a team, and the importance of a healthy workplace. This is just a natural progression with completing a master's program. You get educated on the entire gamut of counseling. I know of too many counselors who are good at group counseling but lacking in the paperwork department (and vice versa).

Five Years of Sobriety Should Be the Standard for Working with Addicts

People get sober and they want to become counselors. In the state of Minnesota, you can practice as a LADC with two years of sobriety. The big problem with this is that two years of sobriety is not nearly enough to get a handle on your recovery. Counselors get jobs in the field and use the group setting as an arena to deal with their own issues. I have seen it repeatedly where counselors get hired by an agency and then come in and make it all about themselves. It is a sick thing to witness. Some stop working their own recovery program almost simultaneously after achieving their goal. They become dry drunks, per se, and become angry, indignant, stagnant "pseudo-professionals." They stop growing, and the goal is continual personal growth. Five years should be the standard set by all licensing boards, as this would give the student in recovery ample time to work through bachelor level courses, get a four-year degree, and intern, while working a daily recovery program. Ask twenty-year sober people what they knew about recovery at two years and the answer is next to nothing. It takes time, and people are coming into the field and doing more harm than good. It creates harm, plain and simple.

Outdated Methods

Treatment methods used today have started to change, but many facilities use outdated methods and charge thousands of dollars. They herd clients into twenty-eight-day inpatient treatment facilities, and many do not even set up aftercare services for clients. Clients get in there, work a few of the steps, and then leave before they have one month of sobriety. Many relapse within ten minutes of getting out of there, and others make it a day or two. Insurance companies spend $28,000 for clients to eat, watch movies, attend lectures and "peer-led" meetings, and get a treatment plan that is "one size fits all." In many cases, it is a big waste of money.

Abstinence-based outpatient facilities are fine, but they are certainly going the way of the dinosaur. Obviously, that is the ultimate goal, but with medication-assisted treatment such as Suboxone and Vivitrol helping to save lives, harm reduction became my "go-to" way of working with clients. Ten years ago, clients were not even allowed into outpatient programs if they were on Suboxone or Methadone. Clients were "kicked out" of programs if they had a relapse or two, which is absolutely devastating to them. If people have used drugs all their lives and their brain has created neuropathways that have made this the norm, why do you kick people out for what they have been conditioned to do? I tell clients they will walk away from me before I walk away from them, and for the most part, this has been true. We have to accept progress "outside the box" and understand that for some, harm reduction is the best it is going to get. Recovery is way more than about using or not using—it is about improving the overall quality of life.

The paperwork required to do this job is insane. A counselor with a larger caseload needs to work a minimum of sixty hours per week to complete the paperwork and then find time to meet individually with clients. Companies force counselors to complete four to six assessments weekly, leaving little time for preparing for groups, completing individual sessions, and then completing all the paperwork that is required by Rule 245G. The burnout rate for counselors is about three years. I made it twelve years, but the job affected my recovery, my life balance, and my overall life. Saturdays at the office completing paperwork is a must if you don't want to drown. If the DHS wants to keep good LADCs, they will wake up and make some changes to this broken-down, pathetic system. They have been making promises for years, such as reducing paperwork, eliminating multiple set-asides, etc. Nothing happens. It is a façade put on without follow-through.

Set-Asides and the DHS As a Whole

Completing set-asides in the state of Minnesota is common for people in recovery who have criminal records and then go back to school, and my case was no different. I accumulated five DWIs from 1987-2004, and the last one was a whopper—my first felony. I have had to complete "set-asides" every time I switch jobs, and with my offense being over eighteen years old, I will continue to have to do this until March of 2023 (fifteen years after being off paper). I have had to complete nine of these since 2011, and in my humble opinion, the people at DHS could simplify this system. My rehabilitation "jacket" at DHS must be 500 pages long. People have told me they will not leave their jobs because they do not want to relive their mistakes over and over again. This system is ridiculous and a way to continue to stigmatize people in recovery. I have waited over one year at a place of employment for DHS to set my disqualifying offense aside. As a matter of fact, I had just put in my notice when it came through. If the set-aside is unsuccessful and they say no? I have just spent one year working with a vulnerable population, and now I am told I have to leave my job. The damage done to certain clients who feel "abandoned" yet again is traumatic and causes harm. One of my best friends (Chris M.) was allowed to work at a sober home as a maintenance man for eleven months before the company received a letter from DHS stating that he must be removed immediately from the facility because of his background check. He was over five years sober at the time. He was absolutely crushed. He soon relapsed after this and died of a heroin overdose in 2018. In my opinion, part of this is on the DHS. Waiting for one year to get a "set aside" back has been common practice, as it happened to me twice. It is a very unhealthy and dangerous practice to allow someone to work and then rip the job right out from under them.

The Auditing Process

Nothing evokes more terror in some of the places I have worked than the DHS audit. They send someone down to audit charts to ensure compliance, which I totally understand, because of the fact that insurance companies are being billed for a lot of money. However, the way this is done is brutal and has spread a level of fear in every place I have worked. Part of this is that many counselors are behind on their paperwork. This has involved counselors pulling "all-nighters" to attempt to get into compliance. When the auditor does show up, everyone walks around on eggshells for two or three days, and it is very uncomfortable. I have seen about five audits done and only have personal experience with two. They were a horror show both times.

The two audits that were done by the Department of Human Services at the place where I was Treatment Director were in 2017 and 2021. These audits should bring some insight into the kind of "profession" I work in. I already mentioned the grievances that were filed against me in 2017 to the DHS, who sent down one of their investigators to complete the audit. She was not a happy person, and this has been confirmed by several other agencies (and multiple people) who have her as their facility auditor. She was cold and callous, accusatory, and emotionless. In 2021, she completed a virtual audit because of COVID. In fact, they were scheduled to complete an audit in 2020, but they were working from home due to COVID. One of my counselors sent a check to the Board of Behavioral Health for her temporary license, and they cashed it but then took four months to activate the license. DHS tried to punish her and the agency for something that was not her fault, stating that she provided services between internship and licensing without a license. However, the BBHT cashed the check, which means the license should have been activated. The DHS doesn't care if you are working with a heroin addict that has been shooting up for the past six months and is sitting in your office ready for MAT and treatment. They want that addendum sent NOW. Anyway, they "surprise" us by stating that they are starting their "virtual" audit on a Tuesday. From that point until the end of work Friday, she sent hundreds of emails to the agency, asking for documentation. She was very cold once again, and the person I put in charge as the "direct contact agent" with the auditor was biting back tears of frustration by the end of it. My time with DHS has been a miserable existence, as evidenced by the incredibly slow process in completing set-asides (remember my friend Chris), the nine set-asides that I have had to fill out, their intrusive visits to audit, which disrupt the weekly flow, but most importantly, the way they treat people. I was taught that we are to treat people in a manner that we would like to be treated, and even if you don't like someone, play nice in the sandbox. This auditor has LADC in her credentials, but it is very obvious that she has never done one day of LADC work in her life. The way she comes off is akin to a prison guard at Alcatraz back in the day (or so I would assume). This is another part of working in this field that is unsavory and sickens me.

When the DHS is done with their audit, they come back at you about thirty days later with what is known as a "corrections order." This is the laundry list of things that need to be cleaned up going forward. It consists of "correcting" personnel files, client documentation, and policies and procedures. It also states whether anything is considered potentially harmful to clients, which usually draws a face-to-face visit. When you read the corrections order, make sure you are in a good mood because you will laugh or cry at some of the absurdities they want you to "correct." For example, we had never taken pictures of clients where I used to work. I see this happening in some places, but we just don't do it. However, one of the things we got dinged for is that we did not tell the clients why we are taking their pictures. I am working with people who are shooting heroin AND methamphetamine daily, and I have to document that even though we do not take their picture, I have to tell them why we are? This is so over the top ridiculous. They are so out of touch with treatment and recovery, and I have to stop everything I am doing to respond to their inquiries. It is just a head scratcher. Very good counselors have left the field because of the massive amounts of paperwork, which is required by DHS.

"Come Back When You Get Insurance"

Those ill-fated words came out of the mouth of the front desk administrative assistant at one of my previous places of employment. The waiting period for people to get help in this state is mind-boggling, and has caused many deaths, in my opinion. There is a "window of opportunity" for clients when they find the courage to come in for help. Some of them are not thinking about how to pay, as they have not been thinking for years. They just know that they need some help and find the strength to walk in the door or make a phone call. This window of opportunity usually lasts about one hour to one day, so when someone walks in the door, they have to walk out with some hope. If they don't, they could be using within minutes. This is just the way it goes. People who come in for help do not want to be told that they will have an assessment appointment four weeks out. They want some semblance of a plan, and they want to talk to a human being. Unfortunately, where I live, most places (and almost every place that I have worked at) won't even talk to a client unless they have insurance. This means they cannot speak to a counselor, make a plan, or set up a time to come back. So...if the client does not have insurance, they are sent out of the door with vague instructions on how to get it. They will get frustrated, and they will get high. We have to take the time to sit down with them for ten minutes, at least, and get them set up with a recovery coach, or call the county for them, or give them a business card with a phone number on it, or give them a list of meetings in the community, or a resource for housing for the homeless. Something!!! Passing the buck is just so lazy and unethical. I cannot stand seeing it, but unfortunately, this is the norm. Nothing is for free, which is why I would "scholarship" clients, do some free assessments, and take the time to meet with them when they came in to see me. I have gotten so many cards and thanks from clients who stated, "Thanks for not turning me away." This is not a job for "clock punchers." More people need to prioritize immediate interventions of some sort, and if you are reading this and you do this, God bless you.

Minnesota: Land of 10,000 Treatment Centers and Unprepared Counselors

To get into the field of addiction counseling, one either has a history of alcohol and drug abuse, a family member has a history of alcohol or drug use, or a person thinks "it would be cool" to work with alcoholics and drug addicts. I just cannot grasp any other reason why someone would want to get into this field. Once a student finishes the courses (six in the state of Minnesota), they work to secure an internship opportunity, and once approved, they are at the mercy of the facility and their supervisor. Counselors are busy, especially at places that are "cash cows," meaning money trumps the quality of counselors. Trust me; there are plenty of them. One local well-known facility tried to hide the fact that an intern was having a sexual relationship with a client, until someone finally made the decision to report it. People who are sick in the field are training young people, and this creates a domino effect in counseling. This is a problem all over the state, with many treatment centers and many job openings. People are looking to fill spots with bodies, and quality, ethical, professional counselors either find jobs as treatment directors or go back to school to get additional licensures to get out of addictions all together. You get what you pay for, and new counselors in the field are being offered $18.50 per hour fresh out of a completed 880-hour internship. This is peanuts when you look at the huge amount of work that institutions force down people's throats. Burn-out ensues, as there is also a large degree of stress in this population. Taking on an intern should be looked at as a privilege, not a liability. I love to teach, so I have worked with over twenty interns in the last decade, and they are all gainfully employed in the area as counselors. However, many agencies take on interns, but do not invest in them and then throw them to the wolves. It is shameful. What you get is a watered-down field, as there are too many treatment centers and not enough quality counselors. The treatment centers are looking to make money over giving quality care, and as a result, you have this "whack-a-mole" effect, where clients just pop up all over the place in treatment centers but are not getting well. One of my former clients watched all three Shrek movies on a Saturday at inpatient treatment, while his insurance shelled out $1,000 that day for the "treatment" he received. Companies buy out treatment facilities and turn them into money-making machines at the expense of addicts not getting well. A twenty-eight-day residential treatment facility normally does not have counselors that work weekends, so in many places, you really only get twenty days of programming, as the weekends are spent watching television, playing cards, using their phones, and sleeping. This idle time defeats the entire purpose of residential programming, as boredom and idle time are common relapse triggers for clients after residential completion. If your insurance runs out after fourteen days, you are brought into an office and are told you have to pay cash or you have to leave. I can't imagine the anxiety that must induce in clients.

Court-Ordered Clients—
A Solution

If you have been an addictions counselor, you probably understand that many of the clients that come into residential and outpatient programs are court-ordered by a judge after they have been convicted of a drug-related crime such as DWI, drug possession, drug sales, etc. At some of the places I have worked, court-ordered clients have approached ninety percent of their total population. Many of these clients are resistant to change and are complying with the requirements of their court disposition just to avoid getting locked up. Some are disrespectful and rude, and take it out on the counselor. This becomes one of the burdens in this profession, as many of these clients do not want to be there and also play their side games while in treatment. It is very common for people to use drugs and alcohol in outpatient programs (and residential programs), as many programs do not provide urine screens (at my first outpatient program, several of my treatment peers would drink with me after treatment and attend the bar I was working at and drink there on weekends). I have known court-ordered clients to have been in twenty-five-plus programs and are still using drugs. State-funded insurance such as UCare and Blue Plus have paid for all of this as well, which means the taxpayer is paying for it. One potential solution for these artificially motivated people is to stop ordering them to get an assessment and attend programming, as this is how many treatment programs keep their doors open. Give offenders a choice of attending or not, or if they have had multiple stabs at treatment, find other ways to dole out sanctions. Community work service, volunteering at homeless shelters, or sentencing them to jail, etc., would be better than sending these people off to "treatment number twenty-eight." This would also close down some of the treatment centers that make their living off resistant clients who do not want to get well. This might sound harsh, but the current way of doing this is ineffective where I live. There are simply too many treatment centers and not enough quality counselors. In the county where I work, there were four outpatient programs when I started in 2012. Since then, five more places have opened, so there are more choices now. However, the quality of counselors has gotten "watered down," with many programs running groups with facilitators having associate degrees. If you lessened court-ordered treatment, some of these places would be forced to rethink their treatment strategies, as ninety percent of their clients are artificially motivated and are doing it because "they have to."

Teaching Learned Helplessness
and Using Telehealth

One of the recent trends in outpatient programming is to give free housing to clients that choose to go to their outpatient program. The clients who make this choice have to attend four hours of programming per day, right in the middle of the workday. This way, clients cannot work, as they are required to make their daily groups, and for the past two years, most of these have been facilitated using Telehealth. The client wakes up, sits in bed, logs in, and attends programming in their pajamas. This form of "treatment" was the answer to the pandemic, and it has been a disaster, in my opinion. Most addiction treatment utilizes group therapy for their platform, and to do this at home in their bed is basically useless, in my opinion. Paying for their housing is another terrible decision by treatment centers, as it promotes learned helplessness, which has always been a problem for many clients. People in recovery need to learn to motivate themselves and build self-esteem, and in an outpatient setting, finding employment is a good way to build self-worth. This "freebie" housing ploy is a straight money grab, as the state insurances get billed for over twenty hours per week of programming for four months, effectively paying for the client's housing. Artificially motivated clients (court-ordered) get the chance to sponge off the housing component, manipulate the counselor through a computer screen, and complete "treatment number twenty" while remaining high. When a program offers free housing for day treatment, which is five days per week, a person cannot find structure in their lives, which hinders their ability to socialize, earn a paycheck, and garner self-worth. I have had several clients come to my program after being in a program that operates through Telehealth, and what they learned there is a continuance on how to sponge off the system. They have no self-worth and struggle to find the motivation to do anything. They have idled around for the past five months, getting on their computers to log into treatment from their own beds. Wow!!! When a "pay for housing" treatment program moved to Rochester, I had not heard of them at all. However, it appears fairly obvious to me these free housing beds are simply "holding pens" to pad treatment rosters. Adding Telehealth to the free housing is a disastrous combination. Telehealth is such as waste of taxpayer money when it comes to doing outpatient treatment. People on Zoom are leaving the meeting "room" for an hour to run to the store or walk their dog. They are drinking while in the meeting, and there is no connection with their peers. It is a train wreck. If people want to get well, they call a program that operates face-to-face. If they want to appease their probation officer, they utilize Telehealth services.

High-Cost Residential Treatment
Should Be a Last Resort

The amount of money the state spends on treatment is absolutely asinine. There were many clients in my long-term program who have had between twenty to thirty treatments, many of them residential. The probation department in Olmsted County is not jailing addicts anymore, as they don't believe in the punitive sanction for people who have substance use disorders. Clients are being allowed to use freely, and there are no sanctions for ongoing relapsing, except "get an assessment and go to inpatient treatment." The problem with this is that research states there is no benefit to inpatient vs. outpatient treatment. Think about this: A client gets into a twenty-eight-day spin dry (these are vacations after one or two times), which costs roughly $30,000. They are in a controlled environment, where they are robotically sent from group to group for a month, not making any of their own decisions. It's akin to living in a human "cocoon," protected from the outside world. They get out, go to a halfway-house or somewhere with "free" sober housing, and continue on with programming. Three months later, they relapse and start the process all over again. That is probably $40,000 for this client. Now rinse and repeat ten times, and you get roughly $400,000. That is the typical client that I work with. Now, imagine this: A client goes to a long-term residential program, which can last up to thirteen months. That is a huge investment by the facility and a huge investment for the client. You would think after completing a program of that length that any further probation violations, etc., would be dealt with by incarceration. NOPE. I worked with a client ten years ago who was twenty-two years old and was in treatment with me for about eight months. Ten years later, he has completed two long-term inpatient programs, completed drug court, and has at least twenty treatments under his belt. Where is he right now? Another treatment. The state has spent probably $1.5 million on him, and he is still going to treatment after treatment. However, because he has made the decision to become a CRI (confidential, reliable informant), he was given yet another chance. As a person in long-term recovery, I scoff at this, as this individual is running around this city, basically "snitching" on drug dealers and addicts, and because of this, he has been given a "free ride," per se, regarding his criminal behaviors and ability to use with minimal consequences.

Drug Addict Informants and their Effect on People in Early Recovery and Treatment

There are informants in every big city, and they bring down the big fish. It is not my place to tell you what is right and wrong regarding confidential, reliable informants, law enforcement, and how they do their job. I can tell you how it affects the drug-using population where I live and how it affects treatment where I live. Here is a typical scenario: An addict with a criminal background picks up new charges (let's say a drug court graduate) and gets booked into jail. While they are sitting in jail waiting for bail, someone comes in and asks them to become an informant for reduced charges (or dropped). This gets the ball rolling. If the person sits in jail for a long period of time, they told them no, and are possibly sent to prison. If the person with felony charges is out on the street in the next day, they may have said yes. In the community where I live, people in active addiction run into me and talk to me all the time. They all know who the informants are. They don't like them and stay clear of them. Many informants are drug addicts as well, and they are put in danger as they are allowed to use, and still "tell on people." There is still the addict/criminal code regarding "snitches," and it is not good. The informant might get arrested, but they are released in twenty-four hours. I know of around ten informants in Rochester who are active addicts, and they get the free ride. They get to use, get people in trouble, and not get in trouble themselves. If they ever need treatment, they will not come to me. I cannot put an active CRI in a treatment group with people who have been snitched on in the past. It creates group derision. I have seen it happen.

PART IV

What Colleges Should Be Teaching Counselors

Tools and Essentials for Counselors in Recovery

This field can be brutal for those in addictions recovery, due to the stress, the long work hours, and the work itself. I want to provide some tips for those in recovery that make the decision to get into this profession, as the coursework in school is very minimal in this area. In my opinion, there should be a required course about self-care, boundaries, paperwork, and the person in recovery. It is that important. I have seen too many counselors who come into this profession unprepared for the rigorous challenges of paperwork, working with sick people, working with co-occurring disorders, and providing evidence-based methods to help those under their care. What happens is simple: Boundaries are crossed, ethics are breached, and self-care is neglected. The group room becomes a place where counselors who haven't taken care of their personal issues utilize the group for themselves, which is dangerous and unethical. Counselors start to slack on their own programs, which brings back those nasty character defects, rendering themselves useless. What comes out of this is counselor burnout, and counselors become very sick, pouring from an empty cup, and causing harm. I have seen counselors cross the lines regarding boundaries, and once that happens, there is no turning back. In the community in which I work, I have seen counselors relapse, have sex with their clients, use drugs with their clients, try to hide the atrocities, commit new crimes, give medications to their clients, store medications for their clients, turn on other counselors, and create an unhealthy workplace for everyone else in it. One of the outpatient providers that filed a grievance against me stored medications for several clients, including Xanax. They did not have the licensure to do this. This is very hypocritical, wouldn't you say? Counselors have to be prepared before coming into this field, and sadly, many begin internships and get no supervision. They are rushed into the field and are running groups within two weeks of starting. They end up doing the counselor's job, and the counselor does not teach them how to be effective in this field. In the second half of my internship, I was running the groups, and the supervising counselor was sitting in her office trying to get caught up on paperwork. This happened regularly in most of the places I worked. The following are essential for counselors in recovery if they want to last in this profession. I have been working as a LADC in Rochester since 2012, and I know very few counselors here that have been doing this that long. If I had known some of these things coming into the profession, I would have been better able to brace myself for some of the sticky situations that happen, and I would have been more vigilant and protective of my practice early on.

1. KEEP WORKING A STRONG RECOVERY PROGRAM

I built a routine in my early recovery of attending weekly twelve-step meetings and working with a sponsor. I utilized what I call daily deposits, which consist of a daily meditation reading, prayer, physical exercise, improved diet, *Big Book* reading, meetings, and working with a sponsor. I call them deposits because you never know when you are going to have to take out a recovery "withdrawal." The more deposits you make, the better equipped you are to make that withdrawal when needed. I turned my daily routine into habits, so when I was hired as a counselor, it never crossed my mind to stop what had been working for so long. My routine had become a ritual, and it has sustained me to this day. Too many times, people in recovery reach their goal of becoming a counselor, and they stop working their own programs. I have found that I needed to work a stronger program once I became a counselor due to the intensity of the profession. When people stop working their own recovery program, they can easily start using the group to sort out their own problems, which cheats the clients. They can also become very sensitive to feedback, which is a character defect with which many people in recovery struggle. DON'T STOP WORKING YOUR RECOVERY PROGRAM. WORK A STRONGER ONE. This would include finding time to continue to incorporate daily deposits into your recovery bank. They will save your ass. I recently spent two straight years working on steps six and seven with my sponsor, and this culminated in the most personal growth I have ever registered. You have to keep growing and remain teachable. This means clinical supervision. Demand weekly group clinical supervision meetings and monthly individual supervision. Compassion fatigue is real, and there is nothing worse than a counselor who is burned out and "empty."

2. DON'T TAKE EVERYTHING PERSONAL

I am guilty of this one, as people in early recovery often have a tough time with taking constructive criticism. I have worked in two places where I felt like my background and history of addiction were taken advantage of when I asked for raises or advocated for myself. There has to be a level of acceptance and the ability to look at things from both sides. I have to always look for my part, and this means I have to continue to be teachable. There are going to be co-workers that you do not like, and there are going to be performance reviews that are going to disturb you. You are going to feel attacked. Take these situations to a sponsor, meeting, pastor, or mentor. Don't sit with them. I recently had a performance review based on my peers, and I was absolutely shocked as to what one other person thought of me. This poor peer review cost me a $10,000 raise, which is a big deal in this profession. My first reaction was to confront all of the confidential reviewers, and my second reaction was to go "bull in a china shop" all throughout the facility. Both would have been poor choices. Instead, I talked to people outside of work that are my confidants, and they helped me see my part in it, which helped me make an informed, healthy decision. Going back to point number one, it is the daily recovery deposits that build the routine, which build the habits, which build the self-discipline and mental toughness. I was pissed off and felt vengeful and resentful, but after talking to people about this, there was a sense of calm, as today I have choices. Choices are absolutely beautiful.

3. SUPERVISION – WORTH MENTIONING TWICE

I was required to meet with a clinical supervisor for two years AFTER completing my master's degree and internship for my Licensed Professional Clinical Counselor (LPCC) license. Prior to this, I was able to meet weekly with some veterans in the field that were in recovery, as I wanted to continue personal growth. This is something that you may or may not have in the facility in which you work. For me, as a Treatment Director, Clinical Supervisor, and counselor, I didn't have one. I went outside the facility to meet with someone who knows more than me, as I have never had pretended that I know all the answers. The biggest asset I can state about having a clinical supervisor is that it gives you a different perspective, a different set of eyes. This is paramount for continued growth. There are also ethical issues that come up that need to be ironed out with a supervisor. Stay teachable and stay healthy. Don't work on an island. We do weekly clinical meetings at the agency I work at, and I understand the importance of these. Some agencies neglect this important gathering as it is non-billable, of course. People need to get together and staff clients, talk about crises that happen in the group setting, and ask questions. Clear the air with disgruntled workers to stay healthy as an agency. Communicate!! The team is important, and catching things early is paramount to staying healthy as an agency. Remember in this field that people leave their supervisors and companies, not the job itself. There is so much movement in this profession, where counselors move from one agency to another all the time. Most of the time, the counselors are moving because of bad supervision. It takes a while to figure it out. Stay attached to a good clinical supervisor.

4. TAKE CARE OF YOUR PHYSICAL HEALTH

The biggest asset to my self-care currently is my gym membership. I work out four or five times per week, and this is an amazing way to let go of tough days. Physical health is so important for counselors, whether in recovery or not. If not a gym membership, walk daily, run, bike, hike, hunt, fish, do something. Practice what you preach. If your clients see you talking about this with passion, there is a better chance they will take it up as well. I brought in a trainer at the gym I attend to talk to my group, and he brought in free week-long passes to try out the gym. See more about self-care in the last section of my book on the intertwining of holistic health and music and how it has given me an outlet for some of my character flaws.

5. BE GENUINE AND AUTHENTIC

Authenticity is the biggest character value one can have in the world of addictions counseling. Addicts can see right through superficial sharing and what I would call being fake. That is one asset many people in recovery have—we are, for the most part, genuine and authentic. Authenticity, active listening skills, and showing empathy are three traits in counseling that are invaluable. Many people in recovery (and not in recovery, for that matter) don't listen, and we need to listen to our clients. We also need to look for non-verbal cues and be vigilant when meeting with our clients. Clients tell us a lot when they are in our presence. We need to pay attention and be authentic. This goes hand and hand with passion. Authenticity and passion are so important when facilitating groups. How do you get clients to stay for that long when we are wired for instant gratification? You have to be real!!! Most treatment programs have many similarities, and the curriculums are not that varied. What is the difference maker? Why are there empty treatment rooms when there are a ton of potential clients to fill them? The authenticity of the facilitator is one, if not the most important trait.

6. RUN FAMILY GROUPS AND ENGAGE WITH THE ENTIRE FAMILY

Learn as much about family systems as possible. One of the biggest relapse triggers for people in recovery is the family system. One of the biggest areas that needs to be fixed is the family system. Run family education groups and find a marriage and family therapist to co-facilitate this. You have to treat the whole person, and the family is a vital part of it (maybe the most important part). This is part of the comprehensive treatment approach that is necessary for recovery. It will also give you an opportunity to educate family members on the disease model of addiction, and give them resources. This part of addiction recovery is sadly overlooked. One or two days of family groups in a twenty-eight-day inpatient episode is not nearly enough. This is why long-term outpatient is the best. You get to have multiple family sessions, which is enlightening, as family members offer "an extra set of eyes" while clients are recovering in the community. I have learned so much about family systems through family programming and family education. The only way to get better at this is to practice. Take college courses on the family system, as it is the only way to do this right. You have to know what you are talking about. Many people say they are providing comprehensive treatment, and they ignore the family system. Well-rounded counselors work with families, and that will enhance your overall reputation.

7. ADVOCATE FOR YOUR CLIENTS IN THE COMMUNITY

Advocacy is something that is a lost art in the world of counseling. It has a section in the *ACA Code of Ethics*, but we don't do enough of this. Advocating for people that do the recovery work is such a big factor in maintaining therapeutic rapport. I have been to court too many times to count, advocating for clients that have jail or prison time "hanging over their heads." It establishes "street cred" in the profession as well. The reason why this is so natural for me is because of how many times I have shown up in court when I was getting in trouble with the law, and having no one beside or behind me for support. It was a lonely endeavor, especially because I did not know if I was going to be taken to jail. I did not want anyone I worked with to go through this alone. Now, a counselor needs to get established in the profession first and build confidence, as walking into a courtroom can be intimidating, especially if you are going to get cross-examined by a prosecuting attorney. It is like anything else—you have to put in the work to get the result. Outpatient treatment in the community is something that will require advocacy. I have been burned by this multiple times regarding client relapses, but I have also seen people make miraculous strides toward progress, and they credit the fact that someone had their back when they needed it. This might be the single most important way to build a therapeutic relationship.

In my experience, outside of drug court, I have never seen an addictions counselor show up for court with their client. This matters to clients more than you know. It can also make a difference in the outcome, especially if they are in a long-term treatment program and you have built a "recovery portfolio" for them, which includes clean urine screens, well-done assignments, and letters of advocacy. It shows the client and the court that someone is committed to them, and it shows the court they are more than just their crimes. It is how some people in recovery get their children back as well.

8. SELF-CARE IS VITAL TO THE LENGTH OF A CAREER

The only person you hurt by working sixty hours per week every week, is yourself. There is no award for counselor of the year (actually, there is, but it is a joke), so the key is to take care of yourself. This is the self-care element that many counselors talk about in recovery groups, but don't heed themselves. Self-care is the most important trait for the counselor in recovery, as it is the antidote for burnout. The average career span of a LADC in the state of Minnesota is about three years, according to research articles on the matter. There are multiple reasons for this, as the job is stressful, the pay is poor, and the paperwork is asinine. However, the biggest reason is that burnout gets the best of many counselors, and for the counselor in recovery, this can lead to relapse or far worse. Self-care will be touched upon in more detail in the last section of this book, but it is an important element of maintaining happiness and not getting bogged down by resentments. People also start to suffer with medical problems if they are living with the stress of compassion fatigue and burnout. I started grinding my teeth at night, which was due to bringing the stress home night after night and not having an outlet for the frustration. One of my admired colleagues that has been in the field for twenty-five years states the reason he does not smile is that he has ground his two front teeth down to nubs and it is embarrassing for him to smile. He also had a heart attack at the age of fifty-three, which is my age right now. This had a lot to do with the profession, being in recovery, and not having a good channel for anger. When anger crops up, there has to be something done about it, immediately. If not, the body keeps the score. A company also needs people who talk about this in trainings. I have always looked for colleagues that are not in recovery for help with this, as many recovering alcoholics and drug addicts are notoriously bad at self-care.

9. YOUR IDENTITY IS NOT YOUR JOB

Your identity is not your job; it is what you do. When I ask people what their identity is, almost all of them confuse this with what they do for a living. They say, "I am a Union carpenter." Likewise, many counselors identify themselves as addictions counselors, and that can be dangerous. I was one of them until multiple people told me that I had no life. If your identity is your job, you are in trouble (see self-care above). My identity today is that I am a father, a golfer, a lover of music, a gym rat, someone who cares about his physical health, a spiritual person, a member of AA, and someone who helps others. It gives people more than what they do for a living – it tells them who you are. This goes along with values. You have to have core values to follow, and these are indispensable.

10. ORGANIZATION IS KEY

It is essential to be organized in this profession, as this can be a high-paced field. I make multiple schedules, one at home, one at work, one for the weekends, and one for my calendar. This may seem like overkill, but this job needs organization because of all the paperwork, information, and the dreaded audits that come from the DHS every three years. I have seen a lot of recovering meth addicts struggle mightily with organizational skills because of their brain imbalances and injured prefrontal cortex. Being organized helps in being a professional and in having confidence. Decluttering your office is also a great idea, as less is more (see the piece on minimalism later in this book).

11. THIS IS AN IMPERFECT PROFESSION

Perfectionism is a character defect for many people in recovery. It saps joy from your life, as you have to work very hard to get things perfect and people get out of balance. One of my graduate instructors sent me an amazing email about the "therapeutic B" when I was struggling mightily with finding balance in my life. She states that my work is very thorough and worthy of an "A," but if I spent five to seven less hours per week on my studying, could I live with a "therapeutic B?" My response to her was, "Don't you know I am an alcoholic?" This is a poor response and a poor justification. Trust me; when I interview for jobs, no one has ever asked me if I got a 4.0 in my master's program. It is of no matter. Think about that when you are in class. If you absolutely just must get an "A," then you will probably suffer more due to a lack of time with family, friends, hobbies, etc. I have worked with over twenty interns, and I have to preach this to all of them. You have to be able to give yourself a break and learn from your (small) mistakes.

12. SOCIAL MEDIA COULD BE YOUR ENEMY

Stay away from social media, especially Facebook!!! Once you hit send, you can never take it back, and it is there permanently. Part of a professional's responsibility is to remain ethical at all times, including away from the office. Many people do not get this, and they post stuff on Facebook all the time. This has come back and haunted them, and I know people who have lost jobs. I have found that being off social media has been one of the great joys in my life. I often yearn for those long-ago days when land-lines ruled the household. Social media is a barrier to recovery, and it is also a barrier to new counselors in the field. I have been guilty of being run down on a Friday and thought I sent something to a friend. It was not. It was to the person I was angry at, and I had to call and immediately apologize. She, realistically, could have gotten me in trouble, but we had multiple talks about it, and she eventually let it go. The point of this is that emotions can ride high in this field, especially if you work with a large caseload. You have to maintain rational thought at all times because if you are running on emotions, something bad is eventually going to happen. Stay away from social media. Simplify your life.

13. GET YOUR CLIENTS RESOURCES IN THE COMMUNITY

Alcoholics Anonymous meetings are everywhere (and alternative meetings such as SMART Recovery, Women for Sobriety, Wellbriety, Life Ring, etc.), and many counselors stop attending their meetings after getting a job in the field, as they just might see their clients at a meeting. By the way, counselors should highly encourage their clients to attend recovery meetings early on, as they are cheap, and there is fellowship there. Find out where the good meetings are, and tell them to attend. It is imperative. In my opinion, AA is the last house on the block, and people try everything in their power to avoid them. Encourage them to go. The recovering counselor should find a way to continue to attend these as well, if they have a history of attending. I never want to forget where I came from, and that is why I continue to go. I have met great friends there, and for new people in recovery, sponsors are vital. Encourage community recovery meetings of some kind, as there are many choices out there today. Someone there could also find a person in early recovery a job!

14. DO NOT IGNORE NUTRITION

Talk about nutrition!!!! What we put into our bodies in early recovery is vital. Frozen pizzas, fast food, energy drinks, cigarettes, coffee, and junk food will NOT make a human in early recovery feel good (I know this from personal experience). There has to be talk about nutrition and the importance of eating right in early recovery. Bring in a nutritionist to talk to the treatment clients and staff. Learn the super-foods, and talk about vitamin supplements such as Complex B vitamins, Vitamin D, and fish oil tablets. Do an entire unit on this. Really.

15. STEER CLEAR OF GOSSIP

Stay out of the drama when working in inpatient treatment centers. William White wrote a book called *The Incestuous Workplace*, which details good and bad working environments. It is relatively easy for rookie counselors to get caught up in some of the drama and chaos of politics and passive-aggressiveness that can permeate inpatient treatment "teams." This can fester between counselor assistants (treatment technicians) and counselors; I have seen it happen at one of the places I worked. It was disastrous. I have also seen counselors I have hired that were my interns turn on me savagely (this happened at the last place I worked). Keep your nose down and work with your clients and bring in your treatment director if need be. This subtle infighting can make your life miserable, and people with two years of sobriety can get engulfed in this. If the work environment doesn't change, talk to your supervisor. You might have to leave.

16. YOU ARE A COUNSELOR 24 HOURS PER DAY

Be a role model by practicing what you preach. You are a counselor twenty-four hours per day when it comes to integrity, which means when you get into your car at the end of your shift, you are still a counselor. If you educate your clients on integrity, act with integrity wherever you are. Be kind, be humble, and be grateful. I remember I was the guest speaker at an AA meeting one night and told my story at about two years sober. At this time, it was more about the problem than the solution. Two weeks later, I was stocking the shelves on a late and long Friday at the Dollar Tree, when I saw someone in my peripheral vision. I started my scowl that stated I did not want to answer any question, and this person came up to me and said, "Excuse me. Did you speak at the meeting a couple of Saturdays ago? I just wanted to say "thanks," as your story resonated with me." She then walked away, leaving me feeling about two feet tall. That is when I learned that in recovery, it is the other twenty-three hours that are so important, rather than the meeting itself.

17. HAMMER HOME VALUES AND LIVE BY YOUR VALUES

Compile a list of your values and stick to "the big four," which are four core values that define your character. My "big four" are honesty, authenticity, integrity, and minimalism. Living by your values is useless if you don't know what they are. These four were built over time, and I needed to sustain my sobriety for a while before I figured out the importance of each. Values are something that identifies your personality and how you would like people to view you. Most importantly, it is how you view yourself.

18. WORK IN THE GRAY AREAS

There are a lot of absolutes that people use in treatment settings, such as, "Don't date anyone the first year of recovery," "Don't make any big changes the first year," "You have to go to sober housing," "Inpatient treatment is the recommendation," etc. I prefer to work in the gray areas and think of what the client wants or needs. When I look back at the twelve years I have worked as a counselor, I think that working in the "gray" has benefited my clients immensely. I was one of the first counselors to allow people in my group who were on MAT such as Methadone and Suboxone, when I started an Opiate Specific outpatient group in 2012. I ran a long-term IOP that lasted twelve to eighteen months when people were running ninety-day outpatient programs. I stayed open during COVID when everyone retreated home. It may not make you the most popular person in the world, but your clients are the ones that matter. Think outside the box with your clients, and stay away from "black and white" thinking.

19. PICK UP THE PHONE

So many people have come into treatment, and stated the reason they started at the facility I worked at was because I picked up the phone. You would be surprised how many people call treatment centers and get nothing on the other line. I also have been thanked by a lot of people because I picked up the phone, or talked to them on the way out the door after a twelve-hour day. Remember that this phone call or random "walk-in" might only summon up the courage this one time. Did I mention that addicts and alcoholics are notorious for not asking for help? Help them by answering the phone, please.

20. BEFRIEND NORMIES AT THE JOB

They know how to balance their lives, and they know how to not take the client's problems home with them. Some of the best co-workers I have had are not in recovery, and I have learned so much from them (not all of them). They are one of your greatest allies when it comes to taking care of yourself.

PART V

Some Final Musings

Balance in Work and Recovery

Balance in the professional/personal life is a big challenge and one that many recovering people struggle with. I know I have "workaholic" tendencies, and part of this comes from my inner inferiority complex. Up until about three years ago, I struggled with believing that I was a good person because of my past, my thoughts at times, and my poor self-worth. That has changed a lot for me, but for many recovering people, there is much to prove to the world in this "rebirth" of recovery. People can get caught up in work so much they forget to have a life. Balance is vital, which is why when we do balance wheel assignments in group, I do one too, to gauge my progress. Like I said before (and say to clients to this day), there is strength in the power of the "therapeutic B," which gives us valuable hours for other aspects of our lives. Let's put it this way: When I first started my career in counseling, I was working at least sixty-five hours at my job and another ten at my second job. My Minnesota math skills say that 75-168 hours were spent working, or forty-five percent of the week. When you add fifty hours per week of sleep (seven hours per night), you have 125-168 hours spent, or seventy-five percent. There can be no time for other vital parts of your life, such as recovery, family, physical health, relaxation, and self-care, which are all needed to perform at your best. Once a counselor is "pouring from an empty cup," boundaries begin to get blurred, empathy begins to be lost, and these character defects begin to run your emotions. Mistakes begin to materialize, and these can be very costly. I have had some experience in allowing impulsivity to rear its ugly head, and this has led to some sleepless nights thanks to some stupid things I said in a fit of anger. This character defect stuff is very real for me, and if I am not working a recovery program, I can sicken pretty fast. This is why I have never gotten on Facebook, as I would probably get addicted to it, which would fuel my addict brain, and take away from bettering myself. The recovering addict still has that "more, more, more" switch that is easily activated, which is why it is important to watch out for process addictions, allowing yourself to work sixty hours per week, etc. Once this switch is reactivated, it is hard to turn off. I think embracing a minimalist lifestyle is a great way to work a recovery program, and that has allowed me to value integrity over material possessions.

Minimalism

Over the course of my life, I never had much. I have only owned three vehicles in my life, I buy a lot of my clothes at thrift shops (Savers for me), I have rented a trailer in the country for the past five years, and I don't engage in social media (other than texting). My years of using have not allowed me to ever really get ahead financially, and up until the last five years, I have never made over $60,000 in a year. I was making eight dollars an hour at Savers when I first got sober in 2007 and eight dollars an hour at Taco Johns. I made almost eight dollars an hour at Dollar Tree, nine dollars an hour at Hyvee, and then eleven to twelve dollars and hour at Cronin Home. The first two years of my sobriety were amazing years of a rebirth of sorts, and I was happy, stress-free, and very much invested in my recovery. These might have been the two best years of my life, as far as serenity goes. I did not need much in the way of money as long as I had a dollar to put in the basket at AA. This planted the seeds of minimalism while in recovery, and it was a good combination. I am a big proponent of decluttering, and this simplifies my life. I know you need money to function in society, go on vacations, take care of your family, play golf, etc., etc. However, I learned the value of being frugal a long time ago, and it has helped me survive when I needed to. Now, this has allowed me to stow away money, and keep the bare essentials. I am happy with this way of life, and it is extremely important in how I operate my life today. It keeps me away from the character defects of greed, jealousy, ego, and pride. If I had to, I could leave in the middle of the night and go anywhere I wanted to go, leaving behind every possession other than my essentials, which would include my music, clothes, dog, and laptop (it is much faster to type than write freehand). However, I must note that I did not purchase my first computer until 2013 (or my first cell phone). I prefer the days of landlines, where you had to get up and walk to the phone when it rang. I have never had a Facebook account, and this has allowed me to stay clear of drama and other tests that the social media jackal perpetrates on people in early recovery. I am lucky

I have stayed away, as I am sure it would have been my downfall. I was very emotionally immature in early recovery, and the combination of Facebook and immaturity do not make good bedfellows. I value integrity over things, and that has helped my recovery.

Stigma

As I just reached my fifteen-year sobriety anniversary and the conclusion of this book, I must state that stigma has been ever present in my recovery. I recently sent over one hundred pages to the Department of Children and Families in Florida, as I am defending my good character against my legal record that goes back eighteen years and more. I just wanted to see if I would ever be able to go there and be a counselor, as my background isn't going to go away. They want proof of my rehabilitation. When I get on the Florida Certification Board Website, the first information I see is "Background Check Failed." They use words like "deficient" to describe my current status, as the powers that be dissect the "package" I sent them. By the way, it got sent back to me "incomplete," as they want me to attempt to get the police report from a misdemeanor damage to property conviction that happened twenty-five years ago, where I was put on unsupervised probation for one year and fined a hundred dollars. I have a binder that is full of all the documentation I have had to send the DHS for the nine set-asides I have had to complete. The last I checked, it includes over fifty professional letters of recommendation over the last twelve years, along with police reports, typed letters of my rehabilitation, ten background checks, etc., etc. The stigma of addiction and its consequences are very real. In the city in which I work, which is well over 100,000 souls, I work with many professionals, including corrections agents and police officers. I know that when they look at me, some of them still see a criminal. Some of them never forget, and that is sad. No matter how many years helping others, how many licenses, or how my reputation has grown in the field, I am still a criminal. It is hard to help people get and stay sober when people cling to their past, as doors that have been shut remain shut. The consequences of my addiction have not gone away. They are smoldering under the next background check. There is a man in Minnesota named Randy Anderson that understands this as well or better than me, and he is a huge advocate for people in recovery who deserve second chances, but are smothered by their past. He is the epitome of what true recovery is, and fights for the underdogs, much like me. Stigma is real in recovery, and William White might have said it perfectly when he stated, "Most people do not like alcoholics and drug addicts." This is very true, in my opinion.

My Blessing and My Curse

When I think back over the past twelve years I have been providing counseling services to folks, I know I have grown as a person, therapist, and group facilitator. I have also worked with large group sizes throughout, taking minimal time off, and have worked well over fifty hours per week over those twelve years. I have lived in the trenches for the entirety of my counseling career, which has given me a lot of practice and repetition. I have been doing this long enough to know what works and what doesn't. This gives me a platform to share some views, but this doesn't mean they are blanket statements. It also doesn't mean that I am right on all counts. I have a way of doing my job that turns some people off. I am a "type A" personality that does things for my clients first. I never got into this field to have piles of people like me (however, that sounds wonderful). I got into this field to work with clients and to help them to the best of my ability. As long as I am operating with integrity and strong ethics, I do not care what others think of or say of me. I have learned over time that people are jealous of others' successes, and that is all on them. I don't need to apologize to anyone, and I don't expect any apologies from those who don't like me. It is what it is, and I choose to focus on the people who do like me.

The blessing of this job is simply that I have a gift of connecting with addicts in a unique way. I think it is a combination of wit, weirdness, authenticity, honesty, and advocacy. I identify myself as an addict, and I can relate to other addicts because I talk TO them, not AT them or DOWN to them. I am still the guy who would rather talk to recovering meth addicts than sit with a bunch of professionals and "talk shop." I talk the language of the alcoholic/addict, and they know that I am one of them. It makes for an easier time in the group room, as they pay attention, they respect me, and they show up in large numbers. I am transparent in the way I communicate with clients, and they appreciate that. I am here for them, and I don't lie to them. At the same time, I don't adhere to the code that you cannot say "hello" to someone you see at a meeting until they acknowledge you first.

My God, give me a break. This is the trait of being genuine that people can relate to. I have spent time in jail—lots of county time. Over the years of doing this, I have had ONE professional state that this was a blessing. This was a judge from Nicollet County Drug Court. She understood—she got it. For that, I always respected her so much. She knew that these clients would buy into whatever I was saying because I had been there. This creates the connection that is vital between alcoholics and addicts. That is why I go and visit clients in jail. I know what it is like. They appreciate the advocacy and the fact that I didn't leave them behind when they made a mistake. I am still with them, even if it is in a crummy jail cell. This is a rarity. They don't forget that. I don't wish the life and consequences I have had on any other professional, but I have paid my dues. Clients can get behind a counselor who used to dumpster dive for food, and is real. That is my blessing.

The curse is that after ten years, I have acquired a reputation in the community, which means there are a lot of people being referred to my program. I would say that almost seventy-five percent of my referrals come from clients rather than professionals. I don't turn people away. I still have a hard time saying no to people who want help, and this gets me in trouble with my self-care at times. There are many times I have come home from work on Saturday and I have given serious thought to finding something else to do, or at the very least, taking a less stressful position as a counselor so I could just do my job and go home. However, these thoughts are rare, and fleeting. I would not be happy, nor would I feel satiated. Working with this population is very draining, and when you work your own recovery on top of helping others with theirs, you have to find balance, and feed yourself something that fills your cup.

I am currently working in private practice, providing clinical therapy, and facilitating small wellness groups (eight to ten in a group). I walked away from the field of addictions counseling on the last day of 2021. I just couldn't do it anymore. It is now the end of July 2022, and for the past seven months, the two counselors that I took in as interns and then hired, are in charge of the place I started from the ground up. I wish them both luck, and longevity. I am very content with what I am doing now, as I still get to work with clients. I am finding more balance with less paperwork, and am continuing to learn.

As for the future, I am very much a restless spirit, and am always looking for new opportunities. I loathe Minnesota winters, and will, at some point, be looking for a change of locations—perhaps Florida? The beauty of my life today is that I have choices, and choices are freedom. I am not tethered down anywhere, and that is a great feeling.

PART VI

My Holistic Health and
the Heavy Metal Recovery Show

I have just finished a long day working in the "trenches." People have exhausted me, and I feel emotionally drained. As I am walking out to my car, thoughts linger on going home, soaking in a bathtub, eating, and spending time with family. However, my vehicle automatically goes one place first. It used to be the liquor store, but for the past twelve years it has been the gym. This is the tonic for a rough day, and I have gone so many times that it becomes instinctual. I do the things I do not want to do because they work. This is what my life has become today for me. I know what the gym is going to give me, and I know how I am going to feel walking out the door. I walk in grumbling and exhausted, and walk out free of the craziness of the day, and smiling. This propels me there, even though it is the last thing I want to do. Yes, I have learned the art of intentionality and self-discipline through my daily routine, and this has built a habit—just like making my bed.

In order to endure in this profession, everyone needs to have good self-care, which means a strong routine away from stress. I have found this in physical health over the fifteen years of my recovery, which includes weight-lifting, Stairmaster's, treadmills, walking golf courses, and a little OCD. I wear a heart monitor when I work out, which measures expended calories, heart rate, etc. This has been a good barometer of my physical health, and it has been an intricate part of my life. It has become an accountability partner for me. I have had to find out my physical limits and push myself to get the optimal amount of exercise without hurting myself. This has taken a lot of trial and error. I got a trainer for one year, and they helped me get started with more intense training. In the last three years, I have lost twenty-two pounds, and my body fat has dropped tremendously.

This is not to brag but rather, to let you know that I wasted a lot of years of my life, and I want to add a couple onto the back end right now. In order to do this, I have had to push myself. I set goals and do my best to obtain them. For example, in Minnesota, there are months when it is too damn cold to be running around, it is dark for many hours of the day, and people eat "comfort" foods. It is easy to be idle and put on weight through those dark months. I made a goal to lose weight three years ago and pushed myself, hard. It worked. Humans can really do just about anything they set their mind to do. Even back in my addiction, there were so many times I woke up and had nothing, but at the end of the day, I had gotten alcohol and drugs.

Part of holistic health that I try to convey often to my clients is nutrition and the importance of good nutrition in early recovery. Diet is a big part of my recovery, and I watch what I put into my body. This has gotten a lot more important to me over the years, especially in the time of COVID, as our immune systems are needed to stave off this virus. I have found that when I feel healthy, my stress levels go down, and I am at the top of my game. It is also important to note that when talking about some of these recovery tools to clients, it helps if you are involved yourself. It enhances your words when you are taking the action, and leading by example. Holistic health has become as important in my life as meetings and working the steps. I don't need to attend multiple meetings each week anymore, as I am living today, which is what people in recovery should aspire to do all along. I attend one maintenance AA meeting weekly, and it is my home group, that I do not miss. I highly recommend a pattern of holistic health to everyone that has started the journey of recovery, but especially to counselors in recovery that are working as professionals with clients. This gives you that extra jolt needed to get through rough patches. It is practical and anyone can do it. It creates structure and routine, and it will make you feel better. That is a promise.

The Inspiration of All Things Heavy – My "Rock" in Tough Times

I must have been about sixteen years old when I received *Don't Break the Oath* by Mercyful Fate for my birthday. It was 1984. Up until this time, I had listened to a lot of AC/DC, Dio, Black Sabbath, Iron Maiden, Judas Priest, etc. When I heard the guitar chords about thirty seconds in, my hair stood up on end. This moved me beyond anything I had ever heard before. I was absolutely mesmerized. This began my love affair with heavy metal, and I mean love affair. I love all things heavy, and my musical vein has changed quite a bit over the years. I loved thrash metal when I was in my early twenties, and bands like Slayer, Overkill, Kreator, and early Metallica were played constantly. I was into Headbanger's Ball on MTV, and these bands were just starting to make a name in the metal world. When the nineties came, I moved into the classic punk sounds of the English scene, and loved The Exploited, Sex Pistols, and Clash. I went from that into Pantera, Machine Head, and Tool in the 2000's, but I have always reverted back to extreme metal. Morbid Angel was there for me since 1989, and I had my death metal phase with Cannibal Corpse and Deicide. However, for the past ten to fifteen years, it has been black metal that has spoken to me musically. Yes, this is extreme music and there is a lot of controversy surrounding it. For me, I don't care about any of that. I love the minimalist sound, the blast beats, and the attitude. This has been my best tonic for handling this crazy world. I haven't committed a crime for years, and I can partially thank this music for keeping me in check. Over the past 10-12 years, I have seen Watain twice, Morbid Angel five times, Amon Amarth six times, Rammstein five times, Iron Maiden four times (6 times in all), Behemoth two times, Belphegor two times, Mayhem, Rotting Christ, Overkill, Slayer, Shining, Vader, Kreator, Goatwhore, Warbringer, and others. I have had six shows canceled or postponed in the past eighteen months because of this virus, and I have suffered due to this. Extreme metal concerts are the one thing that gives me that danger element that I miss from using drugs and getting drunk. The risk-taking of going to these concerts gives me something that I cannot describe, and I don't expect many professionals to understand. They make me feel alive. It's like my probation officer told me a long time ago when she was putting me in jail again, "You are a risk-taker. You are going to kill yourself or others with your behaviors and so I have to lock you up." I think I have always been a risk-taker, which is probably why I stayed open during the pandemic when everyone else closed shop. This music is risky and controversial, but that is not really why I am drawn to it. Like I said previously, it is for the outcasts, and I am drawn to the world of outcasts. This music fits my intensity and my attitude. I cannot be rebellious anymore, but I certainly can feel that way through the music. I am enthralled and entertained by extreme music, and it has never let me down. It is in my veins as much as my blood. I can't really convey this in a way that gives this the actual effect and feeling that the music gives me. It just speaks to me and moves me in a way that nothing else ever has. I was petrified that after I got sober, this music would not mean as much, but it meant more. There is just nothing like it. It takes the edge off, and settles me down. Someone asked me once about old timers in AA, and I thought to myself, "I wonder when I am doing to be an old timer." However, I quickly dismissed that, as I still have Iron Maiden posters up in my bedroom, so I don't think I will ever get to the point where I will be classified as an old timer. I am too much of an adolescent at heart. This music keeps me young, and there is nothing wrong with that. When I am at a metal show, I feel a part of that community, with the band shirts, the attitude, and the vibe. When the arena goes dark, that is when a blast of dopamine bounces off my skull, which is something I haven't felt since that first hit of crack or that first taste of alcohol. Metal fans who are reading this will understand, but the vast majority will be confused. Don't worry about it—you either get it or you don't. About two years ago, I started a scrapbook of my fifty favorite bands, including ticket stubs, signed memorabilia, and other little gems. It is a treasure of mine, and feels good to look through time and time again. I am including the introduction from that scrapbook because the spirit in that intro is real. I listen to these bands at the gym, and it pushes me to do more. I get lost in the music, and it takes me away for a period of time. Music is a reminder of something timeless, and it never lets me down. I am a very spiritual person, and I believe in God as my Higher Power. However,

I still love this vein of music, and that is part of my duality. Here is my introduction in my scrapbook of the bands that make my life complete.

50 Years – 50 Metal Bands –
A Reflection of a Lifetime of Metal Memories

Words cannot do justice to what heavy metal means to me, as I have been listening to this music genre for over forty years. It started with Iron Maiden at the age of around twelve, and it has evolved over time. I have had "music phases," including punk, thrash metal, doom metal, and black metal. However, no matter the genre of metal, the consistency was an attraction to extreme metal music. I wanted to put my love for music in a book with fifty of my favorite bands, culled through fifty years of dedication to the scene. This is the result.

Extreme music spoke to me early on due to a dysfunctional and very strict family. During the time when I wasn't playing sports, I spent much time in solitude, and found a loyal companion in music. As I rebelled against the authoritarian rule in my household, I found extreme music gave me solace and a place to fuel my angst. When I moved out at eighteen, music was a constant companion, as well as alcohol and drugs. After getting sober in 2007, I found that attending concerts became more enjoyable, as I could actually remember the event. Over the past ten years, my musical tastes have become much more extreme, as I have seen the world changing in a direction that repulses me (I will not elaborate here). I began listening to black metal, a bleak, atmospheric, and grim collection of mesmerizing sound that fascinates me. It is the music of the outcasts, and music that gives me an outlet to vent silently through the dirges. I have spent the past years studying the various forms of black metal, including Norwegian black metal, the second wave of black metal, atmospheric black metal, and DSBM. I love them all. I have been able to see Watain, Behemoth, Shining, 1349, UADA, Mayhem, Rotting Christ, and other black metal bands over the years in intimate settings, and the atmosphere is mesmerizing. I have been able to get pictures with Helmuth of Belphegor and Eric of Watain, which are proudly displayed in this book.

The book leads off with Iron Maiden, as I have listened to them for thirty-eight years. I have seen them in concert six times in three different states. They have been with me through my addiction and sobriety and they have been a constant companion in my life's travails. Each band mentioned in this book includes little pieces of history, including concert stubs, what was going on in my life at the time, favorite songs or albums, and other odds and ends. Enjoy – as always, this is not for sale. Up the Irons!!!!!

Here are the top fifty bands that have moved me in some way over the duration of my lifetime (don't hold it against me): (1) Iron Maiden, (2) Rammstein, (3) Morbid Angel, (4) Satyricon, (5) Misfits, (6) Kreator, (7) MGLA, (8) Amon Amarth, (9) Type O Negative, (10) Burzum, (11) Slayer, (12) Watain, (13) Rotting Christ, (14) Overkill, (15) The Exploited, (16) Mercyful Fate, (17) Taake, (18) Sex Pistols, (19) Behemoth, (20) Belphegor, (21) Arch Enemy, (22) Vader, (23) Bethlehem, (24) Cradle of Filth, (25) Dissection, (26) Tool, (27) Mentors, (28) Samael, (29) Cliff Burton, (30) Ministry, (31) Skeletonwitch, (32) The Committee, (33) Dimmu Borgir, (34) My Dying Bride, (35) Black Sabbath, (36) Moonsorrow, (37) Queensryche, (38) Max Cavalera, (39) Siebenburgen, (40) Nirvana, (41) The Doors, (42) Accept, (43) Shining, (44) Drudkh/Hate Forest, (45) Motorhead, (46) GG Allin, (47) Nargaroth, (48) UADA, (49) Hatebreed, (50) Judas Priest

The Ink Tells the Story –
The Duality of My Existence

I have started quite the tattoo collection, and all of these depict that darkness that I have always felt inside. I have two sleeves covered over the past four years, with twelve different designs. My newest is itching right now, and that is an ancient warlock. Each one of these represents a different period of my life, and how I was feeling about life during that time. Whether it was the Kreator cassette I had with me in jail for one year, the Misfits tattoo depicting my love for their horror movie themes, the Taake tattoo with the chains looking up to heaven, the plague hag, the troll stifling the water nymph, Clive Barker art, UADA album cover, Watain art inside "The Wild Hunt," or the Iron Maiden mascot Eddie coming out of the tree (Fear of the Dark, my friends), they are something that remind me of my constant friend, heavy metal. James Hores from the Six of Swords has done all the work—look him up. He is the master of black and gray. Tattoos have become a way for me to relax, and I feel a sense of peace when I enter a studio. It is like walking into a different world. People have never looked too closely at them, as it would require some intentional staring at another human, but if they did look hard, they would see dark designs and images. I have spent a lot of years in the darkness due to my drug/alcohol addiction, and heavy metal music might have saved my life during those times. The tattoos were a way to reward to myself after getting my master's degree and LPCC. I wanted to commemorate a time in my life that was not all bad, as I had a lot of fun too, attending concerts and listening to heavy metal. It was a hobby and continues to be a hobby. Now I have some of these memories from that time in my life on me permanently, and it fits. That's all I can say.

Epilogue –
Serenity Today and Planting Seeds

Fifteen years ago, on May 25th, 2007, I surrendered the life of booze and drugs when I put myself into inpatient treatment. I remember getting up in the morning and opening the shades, where I was greeted by the serene vista of Fountain Lake. Today is May 26th, 2022, and I decided I wanted to go somewhere and finish this book with a similar vista. I have been notoriously bad at taking vacations, and I have never taken one by myself. I made a reservation at Madden's at Gull Lake in Brainerd, to spend a weekend golfing and writing. I am overlooking Gull Lake, and it is beautiful. There is a woman out there kayaking and a shoreline that breathes serenity. This is exactly where I wanted to be, finishing this book I have cobbled together over the past six years and some change. It has been an experience, as I have written this in bits and pieces when time allowed, all the while getting my master's degree, finishing my clinical supervision, and getting my mental health license. I am now working in an agency where I do more individual sessions than group sessions, but I just love group counseling. I believe I have admitted around 1200 clients over the past twelve years, averaging about a hundred per year. Those are simply crazy numbers. Some have done well, and have followed me around from facility to facility. Some have not done well, but that is precisely the way this profession operates. The statistics don't bear out a lot of success, but they are not accurate statistics. There is more to the picture than the black and white outcome of sobriety or failure. There are a lot of factors at work, and the most important thing is that people continue to try. I know I am not responsible for people's sobriety, as they are the ones who do the work. I am simply a seed planter, and this allows me to sleep at night. My career over the past twelve years has been to plant seeds. I am not responsible for the result, but I plant them with purpose and passion, and people see that. I don't take credit when people do well, and I don't beat myself up when people don't get it. I just plant seeds in the way I believe they need to be planted. Some people respect the work I do, and some people don't appreciate the work I do. That is just life. I used to get bent out of shape when I would hear that someone said something negative about me, or doesn't like me, or is being vindictive. Now I feel sorry for them, and I have learned to pray for them. It works, and it allows me to focus on the bigger picture, which is to help as many people as I can with the horrors of addiction and mental health crises. I have always done things my way, but I have always had the best interest of the client in mind. I am an ethical counselor, but not perfect, by any means. I have made enemies in this profession, which is sad, because all we should be concerned about is helping the client. When a client gets sober, it is a win for everyone, as it creates a ripple effect throughout the community in which they live. I remember a calendar I used to have with a saying on each day, and one of them stood out to me. I cut it out and it sits by my work desk. It is a picture of two meerkats, and it said, "I relish the success of others, because there is so much of it to go around." I am grateful I had the chance to work in the field of addictions for the past twelve years, and I am equally grateful I got out of it when I did. I not only survived but thrived in the chaotic world of addiction counseling, and it also allowed me to tell a story. I hope it planted seeds in your head, and I hope you liked it. If it helps one person, it was worth writing. If you didn't like it, that is ok as well, because I can check another box off on my bucket list. This was important for me to do, as I believe there is a lot to be learned from this story. Over the past six years, I have been writing and editing this manuscript, and as I sat here putting the finishing touches on this, I realize it is never going to be perfect. Neither are we. However, I tried to write a book that is informative, honest, and fair, and that is good enough. So, until our paths cross again, be kind to others, and remember to live life to its fullest. Strive to be better, and never give up. Peace!

Acknowledgments

Thanks to the following people, who have been beacons of light in my life, and have helped to shine a light in my darkness: Gayle Olsen, who proofread the book, and provided the Foreword; Betsy Singer, who shines a light on the "underdog," and provides a media outlet to tell people's stories; Molly, who has tolerated my insolence at times, and provides the voice of reason in our relationship; Nelle Moriarty, who allowed me to intern with her, and then letting me repay it by letting her intern with me—you are a great person (and smarter than me); Naomi Oschendorf, who was probably my favorite co-worker and boss—thanks for being you; Jenine Koziolek, who enlightened me on the importance of the family system in addiction, and gave me the privilege to sit in her family sessions; Mike Frisch, who has been a wonderful mentor; "Z," who created the cover art for the front and back of this book; Mike D., my sponsor; Jenna Christenson, a wonderful person in recovery; James Hores, my tattoo artist at Six of Swords; every client I have ever worked with; and last but not least, my furry animal friends Wattie (RIP) and Penny (still the needy Pomeranian, as always). Dogs have always proved to be superior to humans in my life.

I must give credit where credit is due, as I used a quote from the *Big Book of Alcoholics Anonymous* (4th ed.) about the four horsemen, two quotes from William White, and I stated the name of the book written by Anne Fletcher (Inside Rehab). I also mention the books *Drop the Rock* and *The Ripple Effect*, as well as mentioning Johann Hari. These books (and persons) were helpful in the process of writing my book, and I take no credit for any of their work. Even though I have never talked to any of them, I want to thank them for providing interesting books and information on the field of addiction counseling.

Bio

Tim Volz is a Licensed Professional Clinical Counselor (LPCC), Licensed Alcohol and Drug Counselor (LADC), and Clinical Supervisor in the state of Minnesota. When he is not working with clients, Tim can be found on golf courses, in the front row at extreme metal concerts, listening to intense music, writing, working on personal growth, working out at the gym, getting tattoos, and reading good horror fiction. He has always avoided Facebook and lives a minimalist lifestyle, preferring the company of dogs to humans.